Allergies and Infectious Diseases

Rotavirus Infections

Epidemiology, Clinical Characteristics and Treatment Options

ALLERGIES AND INFECTIOUS DISEASES

Additional books in this series can be found on Nova's website
under the Series tab.

Additional e-books in this series can be found on Nova's website
under the e-book tab.

ALLERGIES AND INFECTIOUS DISEASES

ROTAVIRUS INFECTIONS

EPIDEMIOLOGY, CLINICAL CHARACTERISTICS AND TREATMENT OPTIONS

CARISSA D. ZENI
EDITOR

New York

For permission to use material from this book please contact us:
Telephone 631-231-7269; Fax 631-231-8175
Web Site: http://www.novapublishers.com

Additional color graphics may be available in the e-book version of this book.

Library of Congress Cataloging-in-Publication Data

ISBN: 978-1-63321-442-2
Library of Congress Control Number: 2014943361

Published by Nova Science Publishers, Inc. † New York

Contents

Preface

This book discusses the clinical manifestations of the rotavirus infection. It examines the epidemiology, the clinical characteristics, and treatment options available for the infection.

Chapter 1 – Rotavirus (RV) is the most common cause of severe gastroenteritis in infants and children < 5 years worldwide. In the pre-vaccine era it was estimated to cause approximately 527,000 deaths and 2 million hospitalizations per year among children < 5 years of age. Most of these deaths (85%) occurred in Sub Sahara Africa and in Southern Asia.

The introduction of two live attenuated oral vaccines (Rotarix® and Rotateq®) in 2006 has been highly effective in reducing the incidence of RV diarrheal disease in both industrialized and middle and low-income countries. Interestingly, clinical trials conducted in Asia and Africa have shown lower efficacy of these vaccines. This is supposed to be due to the presence of different RV strains in the developing countries and to several host and environmental factors that could reduce the absorption of the oral vaccine through the infant bowel. Nevertheless, a large absolute number of severe cases have been prevented in these countries due to vaccination.

The introduction of the RV vaccination into the childhood immunization programs has altered the epidemiology of rotavirus infection in some settings. Surveillance data from the United States has shown an alteration in the seasonal patterns of rotavirus gastroenteritis with a 1-2 month shift in the onset of the epidemic peak. Similar data has been reported in Belgium. Moreover, some authors reported changes in age-specific incidence of the disease, with increase of the median age of patients.

Herd immunity has been noticed after routine RV vaccination in several countries. Data of the early years following the introduction of the vaccination show significant reduction in RV disease among age groups too old or too young to be vaccinated, probably as result of reduced virus transmission. This finding could have important implications in developing countries where the vaccine coverage tends to be lower.

Whether rotavirus vaccination drives the emergence of vaccine escape strains is still under debate. Differences in the circulation of RV genotype have been reported. In the high and middle-income countries RV surveillance showed an increased prevalence of G3P8 and G2P4. However, it has not been established whether these observations are a result of vaccine-induced immune pressure or simply reflect natural temporal variations in RV genotype circulation. In developing countries it is more difficult to identify the impact of the vaccination in the strains circulation, due to the high diversity of the circulating rotavirus strain.

An interesting final observation regards the etiology of acute gastroenteritis following the introduction of RV vaccine. In fact in the USA Norovirus has become the leading cause of medically attended acute gastroenteritis in children <5 years of age. These findings underscore the importance of continued surveillance monitoring in countries introducing rotavirus vaccines.

Chapter 2 – Rotavirus infection is a common cause of acute gastroenteritis in children, which can cause severe dehydration and even death, especially in children under 2 years of age. There are many publications on extra intestinal manifestations that have been associated with rotavirus infection. It has been associated with neurological manifestations as afebrile seizures, convulsive status, cerebellitis, encephalitis or encephalopathy, digestive manifestations as pancreatitis and even increased risk of type 1 diabetes mellitus. There are also publications relating to cardiopulmonary manifestations with Rotavirus as myocarditis and pneumonitis and even sudden death. It has also been associated with vasculitis such as Kawasaki disease and others. In this chapter the authors will review all clinical manifestations of rotavirus infection.

Chapter 3 – It is estimated that rotaviruses cause approximately 125 million cases of gastroenteritis worldwide annually. More than half a million of these cases lead to death and a majority of these fatal cases occur in the developing world. Humans are the source of infection and the fecal-oral route is the predominant mode of transmission. The infection shows a seasonal pattern in those countries of the temperate climate, which have not introduced a general vaccination schedule yet, and the incidence in these countries peaks in winter months. This has not been proven in tropical countries.

Standard hygienic and preventive measures are not hundred percent effective. Due to the fact that 10 virus particles is the minimal infective dose in humans, the vaccination is the only measure that offers a full prevention of the transmission of rotavirus infections in human population.

Chapter 4 – The passive transfer of maternal immunity provides essential protection in the newborns. It is well known that the neonatal immune system of mammals and birds is fully competent to mount a primary immune response against infection, developing optimal levels of humoral and cell-mediated immunity. However, it is also known that after birth, newborns are exposed to a great variety of antigens for the first time. The initiation of several primary immune responses to those antigens, which in many cases cause mixed infections and complications, would not be quick or strong enough to overwhelm pathogen replication. Therefore, unless adequate maternal immunologic assistance is provided, neonates have an increased probability of dying after infection with common pathogens. Maternal immunologic assistance thus can provide a critical (though temporary) aid to survival for neonates. The evolutionary process developed effective mechanisms for the passive transfer of both systemic and mucosal immunity from the mother to her offspring. Taking advantage of this natural process, vaccination of the dams has become a well-established practice among veterinary practitioners to prevent neonatal diseases. Dam vaccination increases the levels of passive maternal antibodies transferred from the mother via colostrum and milk intake. This strategy of passive systemic immunity had been applied with optimal results, especially for systemic infections. For enteric infections such as rotavirus caused diarrhea, dam vaccination had been the tool selected to reduce the severity of the disease and morbidity rates in cattle and horses.

A complementary or alternative strategy to prevent enteric diseases has been the oral administration of colostrum replacers and immune milk supplemented with protective levels of specific antibodies. Different sources of antibodies, i.e., oral administration of hyper immune plasma; fluid or powdered bovine immune colostrum, fluid or powdered chicken egg yolk IgY enriched in rotavirus-specific antibodies, have been explored and represent effective immunotherapies to prevent rotavirus diarrhea.

Passive immunity has been documented to often interfere with newborn active immune responses to natural infections and vaccination. In the recent years, the transference of immune cells and other biomolecules with immunomodulatory properties from the mother to their offspring had been described shedding light on the mechanism behind this interference. New adjuvants, antigen delivery systems and rationale vaccines designs to overwhelm or take advantage of the properties of these passive maternal biomolecules and cells transferred to the newborns are under development. This review will address current knowledge regarding the mechanism behind the protective and immunomodulatory effect of passive immunity strategies to prevent rotavirus diarrhea in the veterinary field.

Chapter 5 – Group A Rotavirus (RVA) is a naked virus belonging to the *Reoviridae* family. The virus genome is composed of 11 segments of double stranded RNA. Rotavirus diarrhea is a high morbidity syndrome affecting the young of a large number of animal species. Rotavirus is the main cause of neonatal diarrhea in calves and foals in Argentina and worldwide, strains affecting these two species showed distinct genome constellations. Rotavirus circulation has also been reported in small ruminants as sheep and goats as well as in wild and domestics South American Camelids (llamas, alapacas, guanacos and vicugnas) and old world camelids (Dromedary and Bactrian camelids). The genome analysis of the RVA strain infecting these animal species revealed the presence of a genome constellation specific of the mammalian order Artiodactyla. The present review summarized the results obtained by the authors' group research over the last twenty years regarding the epidemiology and molecular characterization of RVA circulating in different animal species of economic interest from Argentina, compared with the finding in these species reported worldwide.

Chapter 6 – Until 1989 all IgG antibodies were thought to be composed of two heavy chains and two light chains. The two heavy chains are covalently linked by disulfide bonds. The heavy chains consist of one variable domain (VH) and three constant domains called CH1, CH2 and CH3, while the light chains are composed of a variable (VL) and a constant domain (CL) which interacts non-covalently with the VH and CH1 domains, respectively. In 1989 a new type of antibody was identified in the sera of the Camelidae family. These antibodies do not contain a light chain and also lack the first constant heavy domain CH1. The antigen-binding site of these unusual heavy chain antibodies (hcAbs) is formed only by a single domain, named V_HH.

The V_HH fragments are designated single domain nanoantibodies or nanobodies® and represent the smallest molecule in nature capable of binding a specific antigen.

These small and versatile molecules can be expressed as recombinant proteins in different expression systems from bacteria to transgenic animals and have opened a new revolutionary strategy of passive immunity for humans and animals.

Advantageous features of V_HH include their high hydrosolubility, thermal stability (resistance to pasteurization process), refolding capacity, and optimal tissue penetration *in vivo*. These V_HH have proven efficacy as a passive immunity strategy to prevent infectious diseases. As an example of their surprising behavior, V_HH directed to Group A Rotavirus (RVA) inner capsid protein VP6 were able to broadly neutralize the virus infection *in vitro*, independently of the strain serotype. VP6 specific V_HH reduced diarrhea and virus shedding in suckling mice challenged with murine RVA or with heterologous RVA. One of the anti-VP6 VHH induced full protection against diarrhea in gnotobiotic piglets challenged with human RVA and other VP6 specific V_HH reduced the stool output in a clinical trial with male human infants. Altogether, these results proposed V_HH antibody fragments as a promising next generation biological platform for the development of immune milks, functional food and pediatric drugs to control RVA and other enteric infections.

Chapter 7 – Rotavirus infections are the most common cause of infant and childhood gastroenteritis. However, a number of neurological manifestations, ranging from benign seizures to lethal encephalitis, have been observed during the course of the infection. Afebrile seizures following gastroenteritis is the most common neurological symptom of rotavirus infection, occurring in 2.1–6.4% of patients with rotavirus gastroenteritis. Furthermore, rotavirus may be a causative pathogen associated with a spectrum of encephalitis disorders including clinically mild encephalitis/encephalopathy with a reversible splenial lesion, cerebellitis, and acute necrotizing encephalopathy. Furthermore, rotavirus may play a role in neonatal seizures, particularly in relation to the 'fifth day fit'. The epidemiology and clinical manifestations of rotavirus gastroenteritis-associated seizures changed after introduction of the rotavirus vaccine. This chapter reviews the neurological presentation and epidemiology of the rotavirus infection with a focus on rotavirus-associated seizures, potential pathogenic mechanisms, treatment, and prognosis. The authors discuss the impact of the rotavirus vaccine on childhood seizures and possible underlying mechanisms.

In: Rotavirus Infections
Editor: Carissa D. Zeni
ISBN: 978-1-63321-442-2

Chapter 1

Rotavirus Gastroenteritis: Insights into the Epidemiology and Control of Infection before and after Vaccine Introduction

Chiara Mameli, M.D., Stefania Pisanelli, M.D., Dario Dilillo, M.D., and Gian Vincenzo Zuccotti, M.D.
Department of Pediatrics, L.Sacco Hospital, University of Milan, Italy

Abstract

Rotavirus (RV) is the most common cause of severe gastroenteritis in infants and children < 5 years worldwide. In the pre-vaccine era it was estimated to cause approximately 527,000 deaths and 2 million hospitalizations per year among children < 5 years of age. Most of these deaths (85%) occurred in Sub Sahara Africa and in Southern Asia.

The introduction of two live attenuated oral vaccines (Rotarix® and Rotateq®) in 2006 has been highly effective in reducing the incidence of RV diarrheal disease in both industrialized and middle and low-income countries. Interestingly, clinical trials conducted in Asia and Africa have shown lower efficacy of these vaccines. This is supposed to be due to the presence of different RV strains in the developing countries and to several host and environmental factors that could reduce the absorption of the oral vaccine through the infant bowel. Nevertheless a large absolute number of severe cases have been prevented in these countries due to vaccination.

The introduction of the RV vaccination into the childhood immunization programs has altered the epidemiology of rotavirus infection in some settings. Surveillance data from the United States has shown an alteration in the seasonal patterns of rotavirus gastroenteritis with a 1-2 month shift in the onset of the epidemic peak. Similar data has been reported in Belgium. Moreover, some Authors reported changes in age-specific incidence of the disease, with increase of the median age of patients.

Herd immunity has been noticed after routine RV vaccination in several countries. Data of the early years following the introduction of the vaccination show significant reduction in RV disease among age groups too old or too young to be vaccinated, probably as result of reduced virus transmission. This finding could have important implications in developing countries where the vaccine coverage tends to be lower.

Whether rotavirus vaccination drives the emergence of vaccine escape strains is still under debate. Differences in the circulation of RV genotype have been reported. In the high and middle-income countries RV surveillance showed an increased prevalence of G3P8 and G2P4. However, it has not been established whether these observations are a result of vaccine-induced immune pressure or simply reflect natural temporal variations in RV genotype circulation. In developing countries it is more difficult to identify the impact of the vaccination in the strains circulation, due to the high diversity of the circulating rotavirus strain.

An interesting final observation regards the etiology of acute gastroenteritis following the introduction of RV vaccine. In fact in the USA Norovirus has become the leading cause of medically attended acute gastroenteritis in children <5 years of age. These findings underscore the importance of continued surveillance monitoring in countries introducing rotavirus vaccines.

Introduction

Rotavirus (RV) is a double-stranded RNA virus in the Reoviridae family, first described in 1973. The outer capsid contains two proteins that define rotavirus serotypes: a G protein and a P protein. At least 12 variants of the G protein and 15 variants of the P protein have been identified. These variants combine themselves to form different strains. The most common serotypes are G1P8, G2P4, G3P8, G4P8 and G9P8. These account for approximately 80-90% of human rotavirus circulating worldwide; however serotype prevalence varies from place to place and from time to time. The reason for these changes is not still completely understood. In the developed countries these 5 strains cause nearly 100% of the infections; while in the developing countries, human RV strains with uncommon G/P type combinations can be a much more frequent cause of disease. These uncommon strains show a wide variability from one region to the next; studies suggest that the circulation of these uncommon strains is probably due to reassortment between human and animal rotavirus strains.

Every day RV disease is responsible for approximately 1500 deaths in infants and young children globally, and is characterized by watery diarrhea, often with vomiting, fever, and abdominal pain, leading to severe dehydration and hospitalization. The severity of RV infection is age dependent. Although the infection can occur at any age, it appears more clinically relevant in young infants and children. In industrialized countries the most critical pattern occurs from 3 to 35 months of age; in the developing countries the vast proportion of severe RV disease occurs by 12-15 months. The incubation period for the rotavirus disease is approximately 2 days. The route of transmission is via fecal-oral route, but unlike other agents causing gastroenteritis, it is very common for RV be spread from person to person. Transmission can occur through ingestion of contaminated water or food and contact with contaminated surfaces or objects. This could explain why intervention to improve hygiene and sanitation (personal hygiene, clean water initiatives) are likely to have a greater impact on diarrhea caused by bacterial and parasitic agents, while RV continues to cause disease morbidity and mortality. Vaccination has been identified as the only control measure to decrease the burden of RV infection.

Vaccine Introduction

The first RV vaccine (Rotashield®), a tetravalent human-rhesus reassortant vaccine, was licensed and incorporated into the USA immunization schedule in 1998. Unfortunately, the vaccine was withdrawn from the market very early in 1999, after the discovery of a small but significant epidemiologic link to intussusception occurring within two weeks after the vaccine administration.

Thereafter, two new vaccines (Rotateq® and Rotarix®) have been developed and licensed for use in the United States in 2006 and 2008 respectively, and subsequently in other countries.

Rotarix® is monovalent vaccine derived from the most common human rotavirus serotype combination (G1P8) that has been attenuated by serial passage in cell culture. Randomized clinical trials and meta-analysis have documented that the monovalent vaccine is effective in preventing gastroenteritis caused by G1P8, G3P8, G4P8, and G9P8. Further evidence reports that Rotarix® provides partial cross-protection against most other serotypes.

Rotateq® is a pentavalent human-bovine reassortant vaccine; each reassortant component contains a single gene derived from a human rotavirus strain encoding a major outer capsid protein from the most common human serotypes: G1, G2, G3, G4 and P8. Various studies have confirmed that the pentavalent vaccine is effective in preventing RV disease caused by serotypes sharing one of outer capsid protein contained in the vaccine. Studies also present evidences of partial-cross reaction against other serotypes.

Both vaccines are live oral attenuated, no significant difference between safety and efficacy has been reported, so there is no preference for one over the other. Clinical data has shown both vaccines have acceptable safety profiles and are not associated with severe adverse reactions. Although large trials before licensure have excluded the association between RV vaccines and the risk of intussusceptions, recent post-licensure data from international settings suggest the possibility of a small increase in the risk of intussusception after both monovalent and pentavalent RV vaccination. The well-documented benefits of RV vaccination need to be considered: the benefits of RV vaccination have been found to outweigh the potential small risk of intussusception. In the pre-vaccine era RV was the most common cause of diarrhoea. It was also estimated to cause approximately 527,000 deaths and 2 million hospitalizations per year among children < 5 years globally, representing 5% of all deaths in children of this age group. Approximately 85% of those deaths occurred in South Asia and Sub-Saharan Africa, 65% of RV-related deaths occurred in 11 countries (India, Nigeria, Congo, Ethiopia, China, Pakistan, Afghanistan, Bangladesh, Indonesia, Angola and Niger).

The introduction of vaccination has led to dramatic drops in the incidence, morbidity and mortality of RV infection worldwide.

In clinical trials conducted in high and middle-income countries, both vaccines have been demonstrated to be 90-100% effective in preventing severe RV gastroenteritis and 74-85% effective in preventing RV infection of any severity. This data has been confirmed by post-licensure studies with vaccine effectiveness up to 100%. The vaccine also determined a rapid and dramatic reduction in the burden of RV gastroenteritis in children aged less than 5 years. A significant decrease of severe RV disease, hospitalizations, emergency department visits and mortality has also been reported.

In the USA, prior to the introduction of the vaccine, RV caused an estimated 20-60 deaths, 55,000-70,000 hospitalizations, and over 200,000 emergency department visits per year. After the vaccine's introduction in July 2006, a reduction in RV-related hospitalization ranging between 60-93% (depending on the age group and vaccine coverage) was observed. A decline in emergency department and office visits and in the proportion of RV positive tests were also found. Similar data has been reported in Europe and in Australia.

Data coming from middle-income countries provide evidence of a substantial reduction in RV prevalence, RV hospitalization and diarrhoea deaths among children. The introduction of the vaccine in national immunization programs has contributed to a 22-41% reduction of gastroenteritis-associated mortality, a 17-51% reduction of gastroenteritis-associated hospitalization, and 59-81% reduction of RV hospitalization in children under 5 years of age.

Compared with the high efficacy of RV vaccination in high and middle-income countries, clinical trials in developing countries have indicated a lower vaccine efficacy. The reduction of the incidence of RV disease among vaccinated subjects compared to unvaccinated subjects ranged from 46% to 72%. This difference in the effectiveness occurs for reasons not completely understood. Experience with the vaccination against cholera, polio and typhoid fever, has shown that the efficacy of liver oral vaccines can be lower in developing countries. Several host and environmental factors (such as interference with maternal antibodies, high levels of co-infection with other pathogens, malnutrition and concurrent administration of oral polio vaccine) could affect the processing of the vaccine into the infant bowel and impair infant's ability to generate an effective immune response. Moreover, in developing countries a tremendous diversity of the circulating rotavirus strain has been observed; an unusual serotype of RV, against which the vaccine is less effective, appeared to be much more widespread, potentially influencing vaccine efficacy.

However, routine immunization occurs in real-world conditions which are different from ideal clinical trials; for this reason, despite discouraging pre-licensure finding, post-licensure data in developing countries have shown a much greater decline of the deaths due to RV diarrhoea and of severe RV disease compared to the experience in developed countries. Given the high rates of RV infection in resource-limited areas, the use of the vaccine has the potential to dramatically decrease the absolute number of severe cases of RV disease and deaths despite the lower vaccine efficacy.

Studies in low-income countries demonstrate the reduction in rotavirus disease following the introduction of the vaccine. Sentinel hospital-based surveillance data have shown that the incorporation of RV vaccination in immunization program has led to significant reduction of all-causes of diarrhoea hospitalization, outpatient visits and of in-hospital diarrheal deaths. The impact of the vaccination is seen especially among children under 1 year of age. On the basis of efficacy data in Europe and in America, the World Health Organization (WHO) initially approved the use of the RV vaccine in these countries in 2006. Following proof of efficacy studies in Asia and Africa, the WHO recommendation was expanded to all infants worldwide in 2008. From here on, universal infant vaccination against RV is also recommended by the Centers for Disease Control and Prevention, the American Academy of Pediatrics, the European Society for Pediatrics Infectious Diseases, the European Society for Pediatric Gastroenterology, Hepatology and Nutrition and by others international scientific societies.

Effect of Vaccine Coverage on RV Infection

Data from Asian Rotavirus Surveillance and from Hong Kong showed an upward trend of both RV gastroenteritis and all-causes of gastroenteritis following the introduction of rotavirus vaccines. A potential explanation for this finding could be the limited use of the vaccine within the private sector that leads to a low RV vaccination coverage rate. However, studies conducted in countries with limited vaccine uptake such as Spain, Greece, France and Finland, have showed a significant reduction in hospitalizations due to rotavirus infection, suggesting that a non-routine vaccination could also be effective in the reduction of the RV burden. In a more recent Spanish study, where a RV vaccination coverage rate of 38% was reached, Gil Prieto et al. reported a reduction of RV related hospitalization of 43% in children < 12 months of age after the introduction of non-routine RV vaccination. This reduction is almost half of what has been shown in other countries characterized by a much higher vaccination coverage rate (83-84%) such as South Australia and USA.

Impact of Vaccination in the Age Specific Incidence of the Primary Infections

Prior to the introduction of the vaccine, nearly all children were infected by RV at least once before they reached 5 years of age, regardless of living in developed or developing countries. In industrialized countries, severe RV diarrhoea occurred primarily in infants aged 3-35 months, while in developing countries the vast proportion of severe RV disease occurred by 12-15 months of age.

Similar to the results of other vaccinations, in national immunization programs (such as measles, varicella and pertussis), there was an epidemiological shift in the age distribution of RV infections following the vaccine introduction.

Data from high and middle-income countries reported an increase in the median age of patients with RV gastroenteritis, following the routine administration of RV vaccines in the population. A study from the United States showed that the median age of patients hospitalized for RV gastroenteritis progressively shifted from 11 months of age (prior the RV vaccine being incorporated into the immunization schedule), to 20 months (in the first year following the introduction of the RV vaccine), and to 23 months (two years following the introduction of the RV vaccine). Almost half of cases occurred in children older than 2 years of age. Another study reported a reduction of all RV cases in children < 1 year of age from 53% to 26%, with a simultaneous increment of the proportion among subjects aged between 12-23 months. Result from studies in other European countries also supported such a progressive shift in the age distribution of RV gastroenteritis toward older children.

Post-Vaccination Changing in Seasonal Patterns of Rotavirus Disease

Epidemiological data has described that RV exhibits a peculiar spatiotemporal pattern, different from that of other seasonal infections which tend to begin in a major population centre relatively synchronously and spread to less populous areas. On the contrary RV infection appears to persist throughout the year even in a small population, possibly trough recurring infections in adults, showing a specific peak epidemic in winter months. This seasonal pattern is more marked in temperate climates areas where the epidemic peak is during the winter months. In regions closer to equator, the pattern is less evident, although the epidemic peak is still recognizable during the drier and cooler months. The reasons behind this seasonality are not fully understood.

Before the introduction of vaccine, the activity of RV in the USA showed a typical Southwesterly to Northeasterly spread, beginning in the West of the country during December-January and extending to other areas of the country in a West to East and South to North direction. The spread typically reached the Northeast regions during May-June. This typical winter-spring seasonality and geographic pattern has been conserved through the years until the introduction of vaccination. In Europe, a similar pattern was identified, with seasonal peaks beginning in Spain in January and then spreading to northern continental regions by March. In Africa RV was detected year-round, but in most countries a peak is recognizable during the cool and dry months. However some exceptions have been reported: Ghana and Mauritius have revealed a peak outside the typical dry season, Uganda and Sudan reported two epidemic peaks, one of which occurred during the rainy season.

Post-licensure studies from various areas have identified remarkably consistent changes in the timing and the spread of RV epidemic following the introduction of RV vaccination. The vaccine's introduction appears to have contributed to a diminished magnitude of RV during months of epidemic peak. Epidemiological studies from the USA have indicated an overall decline in the epidemic peak, with RV activity below the epidemic threshold, for the first time in 19 seasons.

Whilst in some areas, the peak activity occurred between 2 to 3 months later with respect to the pre-vaccination era, in other areas it occurred earlier. A study from Curns et al., carried out during the first 2 years following the introduction of the vaccine in the USA, failed to demonstrate the typical Southwesterly to Northeasterly spread of RV activity. These remarkable alterations in RV activity occurred rapidly following the vaccine introduction and provide evidence in spatiotemporal dynamics suggesting that RV activity in the USA is likely driven by the rate of accumulation of fully susceptible individuals rather than solely by environmental factors previously reported.

Similar changes in epidemiologic patterns of RV have been reported in Europe and in some middle-income countries. Studies conducted in Europe demonstrated a shift in the onset of the epidemic peak of 1-2 months compared to pre-vaccination seasons. In Brazil, a delay of about 3 months in the onset of the epidemic peak activity was registered.

Post-vaccination data are lacking from developing countries and from other tropical areas where seasonal and geographic pattern of RV is less evident. Routinely collected epidemiological data from these countries are needed to provide an insight into the burden and seasonal changes following the use of RV vaccination.

Serotype Replacement

Changes in serotypes or strain of pathogen can occur naturally due to background fluctuation or selective pressures from vaccine and antibiotic use. Post-licensure surveillance studies monitoring the impact of vaccination on the circulation of strains are important to screen for possible vaccine selection pressure and serotype replacement.

Pre-vaccine data showed that while more than 60 different rotavirus strains have been identified, only 5 different serotypes (G1P8, G2P4, G3P8, G4P8 and G9P8) are mostly associated with the human disease in developed countries. These strains are responsible for approximately 80-90% of the childhood RV disease burden in North America, Australia and Europe. Nonetheless, a significant variation in circulating RV serotype has been reported, with yearly, seasonal and geographic variability. In addition, multiple strains may circulate within the same region and at the same time.

Whether the RV vaccination drives the emergence of vaccine escape strains is still under debate. Some epidemiological studies reported differences in the circulation of RV genotypes after the introduction of vaccination. It has been suggested that these changes are the effect of the vaccine selection pressure; however whether this serotype shift is a consequence of the natural temporal variations in RV genotype circulation or the result of the vaccine-induce immune pressure is not yet established.

Clinical trials and subsequent post-licensure epidemiological studies demonstrated that monovalent vaccine has the lowest serotype-specific immune-response against G2P4. Vaccine efficacy against this strain stands at 85%. Similar data has been described for pentavalent vaccine that has been showed to have the lowest serotype specific immune-response against G3P8. Vaccine efficacy against this strain varies between 21% and 71%.

Different surveillance studies from high and middle-income countries have shown an increased prevalence of G3P8 and G2P4 following the introduction of, respectively, pentavalent or monovalent rotavirus vaccine. Carvalho-Costa et al. identified a national predominance of G2P4 strain in the first 2 years following the introduction of the monovalent vaccine in Brazil. In the USA, rotavirus surveillance showed an overall increased prevalence of G3P8 serotype, compared to the pre-vaccine era. Similar data has been also reported in Australia. Here a post-vaccine increment in the circulation of G2P4 was observed in states which use the single-strain vaccine. In contrast the prevalence of G3P8 serotype increased in the states which introduced the pentavalent vaccine. Although these studies expressed interesting findings, they are limited to the first 1-2 years following the RV vaccine introduction in the national immunization programme. Therefore, caution is needed in taking any definitive conclusions about the role of the vaccine in the serotype shift.

Later surveillance data showed that these changes are transient and they are followed by an increment in prevalence of G1P8 strain, which is covered well by both vaccines. It must also be considered that similar serotype changes have also been found in the pre-vaccine era with periodic strain emergence.

Finally, we need to underline that RV disease caused by G3P8 and G2P4 are usually mild form of gastroenteritis and both vaccines have been highly effective in reducing the hospitalization related to these serotypes. More longitudinal surveillance studies are needed to monitor the possible vaccine-induced strain changes.

In addition, some recent surveillance studies reported the emergence of novel rotavirus strains, possibly due to reassortment between animal and human circulating strains. In Australia Cowley et al. documented the onset of the new RV strain G10P14, probably derived from a strain circulating in artiodactyl transmitted to human. In the USA Geoffry et al. confirmed the presence of the new RV strain G14P24 suggesting a reassortment between animal and human circulating strain. Interestingly Lundgren et al. identified another novel RV strain most likely derived from a reassortment with the monovalent G1P8 vaccine strain. These recent findings underline the need to continue surveillance studies to control the RV circulating serotypes changing.

In low-income countries, less epidemiological data are available regarding RV strain circulation after the vaccine introduction. In Africa the molecular epidemiology of the RV strain is complex; the annual circulating strains fluctuate over time and across regions. In the last five years, the distribution of rotavirus genotypes varied geographically from region to region and from country to country, both temporally and spatially.

Surveillance data from 2007 to 2011 showed the G1 strains were the most predominant (28.8%) followed by G9 (17.3%), G2 (16.8%), G8 (8.2%), G12 (6.2%) and G3 (5.9%). The most common P genotypes were P8 (40.6%), P4 (13.9%) and P6 (30.9%). The most common GP combinations were G1P8

(18.4%), G9P8 (11.7%), G2P4 (8.6%), G2P6 (6.2%), G1P6 (4.9%), G3P6 (4.3%), G8P6 (3.8%), G12 p8 (3.1%). Strains such as G2P4, G3P8 and G4P8, which are routinely identified in developed countries, are much less common in Africa. On the contrary, other serotype which are very rarely observed in developed countries, have been commonly detected in African regions. Due to the lack of data it is not yet possible to conclude whether the introduction of the RV vaccine has a role in this shift or if the changes are an effect of the natural temporal variation of RV strain.

Nicaragua has been the first developing nation to include the RV vaccine in its national vaccine program. A recent study from Khawaja et al. showed that following the introduction of the vaccine the strain predominance varied considerably by season. In 2007 the G4P8 strain was predominant, in 2008 the G2P4 was the most circulating strain, and in 2009 the G1P8 was predominant. These changes were compatible with the natural historical pattern of seasonal fluctuation in rotavirus genotypes. This study suggested that the introduction of the RV pentavalent vaccine did not lead to a substantial alteration of the RV circulating strains, as no new or unexpected strains were predominant in the years immediately after the vaccine introduction.

Finally, this report aims to underline that recent studies have highlighted the increasing role of other pathogens, in addition to rotavirus, causing gastroenteritis in children and infants after the introduction of RV vaccination. Interestingly, Pyane et al. has shown that the introduction of the RV routine vaccine administration was followed by a substantial decrease in acute gastroenteritis in children caused by rotavirus and by a corresponding progressive increment in Norovirus infection. Surveillance data from the United States have shown that Norovirus has become the leading cause of medically attended acute gastroenteritis in children <5 years of age, after the introduction of the rotavirus vaccines.

The Role of Herd Immunity

Herd immunity is defined as the indirect protection of unvaccinated people to a pathogen after the beginning of routine vaccination in a population. It is an indirect benefit of the vaccinations and occurs as a result of the decreased transmission of the infectious agent in the community, preventing the subsequent circulation of pathogens in the susceptible population. Herd immunity amplifies the direct benefits of the vaccination among the population that is not the direct target of the vaccination. Indirect immunity has been described in the past for many diseases and pathogens such as smallpox, *Haemophilus influenza type b, Bordetella pertussis, Neisseria meningitidis*, influenza and, most recently, *Streptococcus pneumoniae.*

Surveillance data has suggested the presence of herd immunity after the widespread use of RV vaccine both in high and middle-income countries.

The rotavirus vaccination schedule calls for completing the series by 32 weeks of age in America and by 24 weeks in Europe. There have been no catch-up programs for older children, and as a consequence, this age group is unlikely to be vaccinated. Interestingly, post-vaccination data has shown a significant reduction in RV disease among children who were too old or too young to be vaccinated. This is consistent with indirect protection resulting from paediatric RV vaccination. Herd immunity has been noticed by different studies from United States, Australia, Austria, Panama, Mexico and El Salvador. The reduction of RV infection occurred primarily in the peak months of rotavirus activities and persisted for more than 3 consecutive years; both these findings are very unlikely due to year-to-year natural rotavirus variation. Moreover, Gastanaduy et al. has recently demonstrated a significant reduction of RV prevalence in adult population similarly to what occurs in the paediatric population after vaccine widespread. This data is strongly consistent with the indirect immunity effect of infant rotavirus vaccination which could be extended to adult population as well.

Data on herd immunity represent important findings. If indirect immunity could be less relevant in developed countries where efficacy and coverage of vaccine reach 90%, it became extremely important in developing countries where efficacy and coverage of the vaccination tend to be lower. In low-income countries a vaccine that provides an indirect immunity could bring much greater benefits to the population as compared with the benefits of direct effectiveness. In these settings, herd immunity could save consistent numbers of lives over the years. Unfortunately data about herd immunity from developing countries are lacking. Considering the relevant epidemiological differences (such as serotype circulation, severity of disease, median age of onset, etc.), it is hard to predict if indirect effects of the vaccination seen in industrialized countries might also apply in low-income settings.

Conclusion

Rotavirus vaccine has reduced the burden of RV disease, hospitalization and mortality rate due to RV infection both in industrialized and in developing countries. If pre-vaccine studies have shown less effectiveness of RV vaccine in low-income settings, post-licensure surveillance data have described a much greater reduction of the absolute number of RV severe infections, hospitalization and deaths due to RV gastroenteritis. Surveillance data from all over the world in the years after the RV vaccine introduction in the national immunization schedule, have reported significant epidemiological changes in the median age of onset of RV infection, in the seasonal and geographic pattern of the RV epidemic peak and in the serotype circulation both in industrialized and in developing countries. Data about herd immunity induced by RV vaccination are now available. This finding could be very important considering the implication of indirect immunity in developing countries where the coverage for the RV vaccine is much lower then what registered in industrialized countries and, in contrast, the RV gastroenteritis is much more common causing the great part of RV induced deaths.

Long-term monitoring will need to continue to assess the effects of rotavirus immunization programs especially in low-income countries, where vaccine programs have recently been instituted. Moreover, epidemiologic strain surveillance is necessary to determinate whether changes in strain ecology change the RV vaccine effectiveness.

References

Assis ASF, Valle DA, Antunes GR, et al. Rotavirus epidemiology before and after vaccine introduction. *J. Pediatr. (Rio J).* 2013, 89, 470-6.

Chetrit E, L' Homme Y, Sohal JS, et al. Group A rotaviruses in children with gastroenteritis in a Canadian pediatric hospital: the prevaccine era. *Can. J. Infec. Dis. Med. Microbiol.* 2013, 24, E1-6.

Chiang GP, Nelson EA, Pang TJ, et al. Rotavirus incidence in hospitalised Hong Kong children: 1 July 1997 to 31 March 2011. *Vaccine.* 2014;32:1700-6.

Cortese MM, Immergluck LC, Held M, et al. Effectiveness of monovalent and pentavalent rotavirus vaccine. *Pediatrics.* 2013; 132:e25-33.

Cowley D, Donato CM, Roczo-Farkas S, et al. Novel G10P [14] rotavirus strain, northern territory, Australia. *Emerg. Infect. Dis.* 2013; 19:1324-7.

da Silva Soares L, de Fátima Dos Santos Guerra S, do Socorro Lima de Oliveira A, et al. Diversity of rotavirus strains circulating in Northern Brazil after introduction of a rotavirus vaccine: High prevalence of G3P [6] genotype. *J. Med. Virol.* 2013 Oct 17. doi: 10.1002/jmv.23797.

Dennehy PH. Effect of vaccine on rotavirus disease in the pediatric population. *Current Opinion*. 2012, 76-84.

Esparza-Aguilar M, Gastañaduy PA2, Sánchez-Uribe E1 et al. Diarrhoea-related hospitalizations in children before and after implementation of monovalent rotavirus vaccination in Mexico. *Bull. World Health Organ.* 2014;9:117-25.

Gastanaduy PA, Curns AT, Parashar UD, et al. Gastroenteritis hospitalization in older children and adults in the United States before and after implementation of infant Rotavirus vaccination. *JAMA*. 2013, 310, 851-3.

Gil-Prieto R, Gonzalez-Escalada A, Alvaro-Meca A, et al. Impact of non-routine rotavirus vaccination on hospitalizations for diarrhoea and rotavirus infections in Spain. *Vaccine*. 2013; 31:5000-4.

Hemming M, Vesikari T. Genetic diversity of G1P [8] rotavirus VP7 and VP8* antigens in Finland over a 20-year period: No evidence for selection pressure by universal mass vaccination with RotaTeq® vaccine. *Infect. Genet. Evol.* 2013; 19:51-8.

Khawaja S, Cardellino A, Mast TC. Hospital-based surveillance and analysis of genotype variation in nicaragua after the introduction of the pentavalent rotavirus vaccine. *Pediatr. Infect. Dis. J.* 2014; 33:e25-8.

Linhares AC, Justino MC. Rotavirus vaccination in Brazil: effectiveness and health impact seven years post-introduction. *Expert Rev. Vaccines*. 2014; 13:43-57.

Mameli C, Fabiano V, Zuccotti GV. New insight into rotavirus vaccine. *Human Vaccines and immunotherapeutics*. 2012, 8, 1-7.

Matthijnssens J, Zeller M, Heylen E et al. The RotaBel study group. Higher proportion of G2P [4] rotaviruses in vaccinated hospitalised cases compared to unvaccinated hospitalised cases, despite high vaccine effectiveness against heterotypic G2P [4] rotaviruses. *Clin. Microbiol. Infect.* 2014 Mar 3.

Msimang VM, Page N, Groome MJ et al. Impact of rotavirus vaccine on childhood diarrheal hospitalization after introduction into the South african public immunization program. *Pediatr. Infect. Dis. J.* 2013; 32:1359-64.

Msimang VM, Page N, Groome MJ, et al. Impact of Rotavirus Vaccine on Childhood Diarrheal Hospitalization Following Introduction into the South African Public Immunization Program. *Pediatr. Infect. Dis J.* 2013 Aug 8.

Mwenda JM, Tate JE, Prashar UD, et al. African sotavirus surveillance network. *Pediatr. Infect. Dis. J.* 2014, 33 S6-8.

Mwenda JM, Tate JE, Steele AD, et al. Preparing for the scale-up of rotavirus vaccine introduction in Africa. *Pediatr. Infect. Dis.* 2014, 33, S1-5.

Ngabo F, Gatera M, Karema C, et al. Can routinely collcted national data on childhood morbidity and mortality from diarrhea be used to monitor health impact of rotavirus vaccination in Africa. *Pediatr. Infect. Dis. J.* 2014, 33, S89-93.

Panozzo CA, Becker-Dreps S, Pate V et al. Indirect, Total, and Overall Effectiveness of the Rotavirus Vaccines for the Prevention of Gastroenteritis Hospitalizations in Privately Insured US Children, 2007-2010. *Am. J. Epidemiol.* 2014 Feb 26.

Pashar UD, Gibson JD. Rotavirus and severe childhood diarrhea. *Emerg. Inect. Dis.* 2006, 12, 304-6.

Patel MM, Steele D, Gentsch JR, et al. Real-world impact of rotavirus vaccination. *Pediatr. Infect. Dis. J.* 2011, 30 S1-5.

Patton JT. Rotavirus diversity and evolution in the post-vaccine world. *Discov. Med.* 2012, 13: 85-97.

Payne DC, Vinjé J, Szilagyi PG, et al. Norovirus and medically attended gastroenteritis in U.S. children. *N. Engl. J. Med.* 2013, 368, 1121-30.

Pendleton A1, Galic M, Clarke C, et al. Impact of rotavirus vaccination in Australian children below 5 years of age: a database study. *Hum. Vaccin Immunother.* 2013; 9:1617-25.

Pitzer VE, Viboud C, Simonsen L, et al. Demographic variability vaccination and the spatiotemporal dynamics of rotavirus epidemics. *Science.* 2009, 325, 290-4.

Rose TL, Marques da Silva MF, Goméz MM et al. Evidence of vaccine-related reassortment of rotavirus, Brazil, 2008-2010. *Emerg. Infect. Dis.* 2013; 19:1843-6.

Rotavirus surveillance: worldwide, 2009. *MMWR Morb. Wkly. Rep.* 2011; 60: 514- 516.

Seheri M, Nemarude L, Peenze I, et al. Update of rotavirus strains circulating in Africa from 2009 through 2011. *Pediatr. Infect. Dis. J.* 2014, 33, S76-84.

Seheri M, Nemarude L, Peenze I, et l. Update of rotavirus strains circulating in Africa from 2007 through 2011. *Pediatr. Infect. Dis. J.* 2014; 33 Suppl 1:S76-84.

Staat MA, Payne DC, Donauer S, et al. Effectiveness of pentavalent rotavirus vaccine against severe disease. *Pediatrics*. 2011, 128, E267-75.

Vesikari T, Uhari M, Renko M, et al. Impact and Effectiveness of RotaTeq® Vaccine Based on 3 Years of Surveillance Following Introduction of a

Rotavirus Immunization Program in Finland. *Pediatr. Infect. Dis. J.* 2013 D;32:1365-73.

Weinberg GA, Teel EN, Mijatovic-Rustempasic S, et al. Detection of novel rotavirus strain by vaccine postlicensure surveillance. *Emerg. Infect. Dis.* 2013; 19:1321-3.

Weintraub ES, Baggs J, Duffy J, et al. Risk of intussusception after monovalent rotavirus vaccination. *N. Engl. J. Med.* 2014, 370, 513-9.

Yih WK, Lieu TA, Kulldorff M, et al. Intussusception risk after rotavirus vaccination in U.S. infants. *N. Engl. J. Med.* 2014;370:503-12.

In: Rotavirus Infections
Editor: Carissa D. Zeni
ISBN: 978-1-63321-442-2

Chapter 2

Extraintestinal Manifestations of Rotavirus Infection

M. J. Carbonero Celis, M. C. Cuadrado Caballero, B. Relinque Macías and F. Argüelles Martín
Hospital Universitario Virgen Macarena, Sevilla, Spain

Abstract

Rotavirus infection is a common cause of acute gastroenteritis in children, which can cause severe dehydration and even death, especially in children under 2 years of age. There are many publications on extraintestinal manifestations that have been associated with rotavirus infection. It has been associated with neurological manifestations as afebrile seizures, convulsive status, cerebellitis, encephalitis or encephalopathy, digestive manifestations as pancreatitis and even increased risk of type 1 diabetes mellitus. There are also publications relating to cardiopulmonary manifestations with Rotavirus as myocarditis and pneumonitis and even sudden death. It has also been associated with vasculitis such as Kawasaki disease and others. In this chapter we will review all clinical manifestations of rotavirus infection.

Introduction

Rotaviruses are RNA viruses (Reoviridae family) and were discovered by Dr. Ruth Bishop in 1973 in Australia, the electron microscope have appearance similar to a wheel feature.

Using the immunogenic characteristics of the capsid protein VP6 7 have identified antigenic serogroups (A, B, C, D, E, F and G) which three (A, B and C) infect humans. The A group which accounts for more than 90% of rotavirus gastroenteritis in humans, is endemic worldwide. Each year rotavirus causes millions of cases of diarrhoea in developing countries, almost 2 million resulting in hospitalisation and an estimated 611,000 resulting in death. The B group has caused large outbreaks in China. The C group have very low prevalence. Groups D and E have been isolated only animals.

Almost every child has been infected with rotavirus by age five. It is the leading single cause of severe diarrhoea among infants and children, being responsible for about 20% of cases, and accounts for 50% of the cases requiring hospitalisation. In temperate areas, rotavirus infections occur primarily in the winter, but in the tropics they occur throughout the year; the difference is partly explained by seasonal changes in temperature and humidity. The number attributable to food contamination is unknown.

The minimum infective dose of rotavirus is estimated at 10 to 100 viral particles. A sick excreted 100-1010 infectious particles per ml of stool. The clinical picture is characterized by an incubation period of 2 days, vomiting and watery diarrhea for 3 to 8 days, fever and abdominal pain. The first symptom appears as vomiting accompanied by a slight feverishness, they are giving 24 hours of the disease and then diarrhea starts, other symptoms may occur such as abdominal pain and symptoms respiratory and rapidly progressing dehydration in infants occur. The stool is usually without gross blood or white blood cells.

Patients with rotavirus diarrhea, benign or severe convulsions, or encephalitis have evidence of rotavirus in the cerebrospinal fluid (CSF). Although rotavirus antigenemia is frequently observed in a patient's serum during the acute phase, the CSF is not always positive for rotavirus antigen or PCR product. The pathophysiological mechanism is still unclear. Although cerebellar disorders sometimes occur as a complication of rotavirus gastroenteritis.

Recently it has been associated with other extraintestinal manifestations such as neurological, digestive, liver, bacteremia or sepsis, with vasculitis such as Kawasaki disease or other rare and sudden death Infections in neonates are generally mild or asymptomatic, but some may present as necrotizing enterocolitis (NEC), a severe form of gastrointestinal disease in neonates and young infants.

Occurs immunity after infection and subsequent boxes are usually less severe than the original infection. It is not necessary to isolate a person who have diarrhea rotavirus or exclude children from their nursery. However, as long as diarrhea and virus shedding (eighth day), avoid contact with healthy children sick.

Neurological Manifestations of Rotavirus

Rotavirus infection is basically localized in the intestine, but rare cases with morbidity result from extra-intestinal involvement. Neurological manifestations occur in approximately 2-5% of Rotavirus Gastroenteritis, these manifestations ranging from mild abnormalities of the state, such as drowsiness or restlessness, severe neurological disorders.

There have been reports of encephalitis, encephalopathy, Reye and Reye-like syndrome, acute necrotizing encephalitis, flaccid paralysis, meningitis and febrile or afebrile seizures.

There is no consensus about the pathophysiology and several theories have been proposed in recent years.

Initially, it was thought that the replication of virus Rotavirus, took place exclusively in the gastrointestinal tract, the association of gastrointestinal symptoms with high fever, hypertransaminasemia, encephalitis and seizures suggested that it replicated systemically.

Rotavirus RNA was detected in 80% of stool cultures in patients with rotavirus diarrhea with or without neurological involvement, just as often the detection of Rotavirus antigen in the blood during the acute phase. However cerebrospinal fluid (CSF) will only be detected in the presence of neurological impairment.

Besides the fact that 50% of cases has been detected the same structural gene sequence in feces VP7 and CSF indicates the existence of a certain neurotrophism.

The theory of virus replication systemically with subsequent invasion hematogenous central nervous system (CNS) is supported by the presence of antigen and the genome of rotavirus in CSF, blood, and stools detected by chain reaction of the polymerase with reverse transcriptase (RT-PCR). It has also been detected in CSF anti-RV immunoglobulin G in some patients with neurological symptoms.

Furthermore, the finding of elevated concentrations of carnitine, and nitric oxide in CSF of patients with neurological symptoms, has postulated the existence of an increased permeability of the blood-brain barrier as a possible cause.

The same way the role of the immune response viremia and the severity of the disease and on protective immunity against reinfection is unknown.

The neurological symptoms that most often come from rotavirus infection are already defined by Morooka in 1982 as a benign childhood convulsions with mild gastroenteritis (CwG).

They consist of afebrile seizures associated with gastrointestinal symptoms in the absence of dehydration and electrolyte disturbance in previously healthy children (Table 1).

Although Rotavirus appears to be primarily responsible for this entity, CwG are not specific to rotavirus infection, have been isolated other viruses such as Norovirus.

In the Asian children population this association is quite frequent, being a well-defined entity. In our setting, the prevalence of CwG varies between 2.06% and 6.4% of secondary Rotavirus diarrhea. The age of onset is between 6 months and 3 years of age, with a peak incidence between 12-24 months. Seizures usually appear after 24-72 hours of onset of gastrointestinal symptoms, but sometimes precede the appearance thereof or delayed until after 7 days. The presentation is in cluster; it is self-limiting short crisis usually in less than 5 minutes but can reach 20 minutes.

Table 1. Defining characteristics of CwG

Previously healthy infants and young children aged 6 months to 3 years having afebrile
generalized convulsions associated with symptoms of gastroenteritis
Seizures occurring sometimes in cluster
Normal laboratory examination results including for electrolytes, blood glucose and cerebrospinal fluid
Normal interictal electroencephalography
Excellent developmental outcomes

It has been determined tonic-clonic as how most common presenting generalized seizures, however Komori et al., reported ten cases of CwG. Nineteen seizures were observed over all episodes. The seizures were mostly brief (within 5 min). However, case 9 had two prolonged seizures: 20 min of generalized tonic seizure with pedalling-like movement and 10 min of atonic seizure. The seizures were often repetitive in clusters (19 seizures/l0 episodes); three patients had only one seizure in their episodes, while the other seven had two or more seizures; two seizures were observed in 6 cases and three seizures in one case. Nine of the 19 seizures were classified as generalized seizures, while the other 10 were partial seizures including hemiconvulsions in two patients, generalized seizures with lateral gaze in 6, and accompanying with pedalling-like movements in one. In six patients, the seizure type changed during the episode, Uemura et al. describe some of the seizures were characterized by loss of consciousness, eye deviation, cyanosis, and no or subtle convulsive movements. These facts imply that the type of seizures is likely to be secondary generalized in patients with CwG. According Li et al., the reasons for the high percentage of generalized seizures found in studies were probably because focal seizures can rapidly become secondarily generalized and no ictal EEG were obtained in all patients.

At first, the absence of family and personal history of epilepsy was part of the diagnostic basis of this entity, however studies have reported a history of febrile seizures in up to 20% of cases and afebrile by up to 6%, which suggests a possible genetic predisposition.

Lab tests, including CSF examination, electrolyte balance and blood glucose are normal. The brain activity recorded by EEG reflects a pattern of normal activity even during crises slowed slightly registration may appear. Okumura et al. determined that the answer to the classic anticonvulsant drugs including combination therapy would be ineffective in 50% of cases. With the growing knowledge of this entity, there are new therapeutic alternatives.

Hayhasi et al. proposed the use of lidocaine, being more effective than diazepam and phenobarbital for seizure termination. An efficiency of 100% is estimated after continuous infusion of lidocaine, however the side effects due to treatment contrasts with the benign nature of the crisis. The use of lidocaine patches proposed by Okumura et al., avoid these side effects, and has an efficiency of 62% may be a reasonable alternative. Furthermore, Eroki et al., after rejecting the use of lidocaine infusion, due to its undesirable effects, proposed using hydrate rectal chloral single dose, and effective for the treatment of CwG, recommending its use in a dose not under 40mgxkg. Once the crisis seriously curtailed, no epileptic treatment or preventive maintenance is recommended.

The standard is the seizure recurrence with a mean of 2.5 seizures per patient being these short-lived. Ichiyama et al. proposed dose of 5mg/kg/day carbamazepine at short intervals of time, showing to be effective in reducing seizure recurrence.

The prognosis is favorable with no neurological sequelae. Even in cases that progressed to status epilepticus, healing was complete after normal psychomotor development.

Children with a history of CwG, with new episodes secondary to Rotavirus GEA seizures again presented with similar characteristics in 10% of cases. However, there is an increased risk of developing epilepsy.

It is important to consider this entity to avoid unnecessary additional tests and prolonged antiepileptic treatments. Apart from CwG, febrile seizures was described after rotavirus infections. Through a study of the characteristics presented in 59 children with seizures secondary to rotavirus (27 afebrile and 32 febrile), Lee et al. defend the value of febrile as independent crisis CwG after determining the following differential characteristics were analyzed: home early after gastrointestinal symptoms, less frequent presentation crisis cluster, and longer the same. In addition, the frequent finding of family and personal history of previous febrile seizures in these patients suggests a different pathogenic mechanism, based on strong genetic influence and neuronal hyperexcitability.

Furthermore, different grades of encephalitis/encephalopathy described after gastrointestinal infection in patients with stool positive for Rotavirus. Secondary cerebellitis to rotavirus infection is usually associated with encephalitis/encephalopathy, cerebellar symptomatology evidenced after a decrease in the level of consciousness which may be accompanied or not seizures.

Cerebellar insult will be characterized by motor dysfunction with impaired fine and gross motor, head and trunk hypotonia, ataxia and tremor of attitude. The most characteristic symptom of this syndrome will be the silence, present in the acute and subacute phase. Cerebellar mutism after resection of posterior fossa is a well-known entity. It appears after resection of tumor at cerebellar mutism persistent variable from days to months post-surgery, usually with persistent dysarthria. The mechanism leading to secondary post cerebellitis mutism to rotavirus infection seems vasospasm outflow tracts of toothed cores via the ventrolateral thalamus superior cerebellar peduncle.

The normal evolution is the gradual standardization of language and motor disorders, and these more recent persistent over time, and may even persist dysarthria and explosive type language.

A brain diffusion-weighted magnetic resonance imaging (BDWRI) revealed chronological changes, marked hyperintensity in the bilateral dentate nucleus followed by hyperintensity in the vermis. Evolution is towards progressive decrease with subsequent appearance of hyperintensity at cerebellar atrophy.

Cases secondary to rotavirus infection in which Rotavirus RNA was detected in CSF cerebellitis described in the literature.

Kobayashi et al. reported on two cases, one with viral RNA detected in cerebrospinal fluid, which also demonstrated cerebellar foci on diffusion-weighted magnetic resonance imaging and residual cerebellar atrophy.

Other reports presented suspected cases with cerebellar signs, although viral RNA could not be isolated from the cerebrospinal fluid.

Reye Syndrome

Reye syndrome is a potentially fatal syndrome that has numerous detrimental effects to many organs, especially the brain and liver. The classic features are a rash, vomiting, abrupt encephalopathy associated with fatty degeneration in the liver. There may be changes in the patient´s level of consciousness, seizures, coma and death. It has a high mortality rate, from 20 to 40 %.

Severe hepatitis or Reye syndrome with rotavirus gastroenteritis in children has rarely reported. The first case was reported in 1978 by Salmi, later, in a review in 203 cases diagnosed as a Reye syndrome in the UK between in 10 years, there were 57 patients with viral infections, with three cases of rotavirus. Some were fatal and some recovered without any sequela. All presents the typical features of Reye syndrome: hypoglycemia, extensive derangement of the transaminases with normal bilirubin.

Reye syndrome has been associated with aspirin consumption by children with viral illness. It also occurs in the absence of aspirin use, so the exact cause is unknown. The association with Rotavirus infection could be caused a cytokine storm, and first activated glia cells in the central nervous system by cytokines followed by liver dysfunction and hyperammnonia which caused acute brain oedema.

Necrotizing Enterocolitis

Necrotizing enterocolitis (NEC) is one of the potentially most serious diseases in neonatal units, which mainly affects infants of very low birth weight, low gestational age, low Apgar scores and perinatal complications. It is a clinical syndrome of ischemic bowel necrosis characterized by the presence gastrointestinal disorders such as tenderness and bloating, it may be as ileus, gastrointestinal bleeding, intestinal perforation and peritonitis. They may have symptoms and signs suggestive of sepsis and systemic shock. It's a multifactorial etiology, both infectious and non-infectious factors. The predominant organisms include Enterobacteriaceae (Escherichia coli, Klebsiella pneumoniae), Clostridium, enteric pathogens (Salmonella, Coxsackie, Coronavirus, Rotavirus) and potential pathogens such as Bacteroides fragilis.

Have been reported several outbreaks of rotavirus infection in neonatal units indifferent countries. Rotaviruses are the most common viral agents associated with NEC. The main reservoir of rotavirus infection in neonatal units appears to be infected newborns, and most of the infection occurs in the first days of life. Preterm, low birth weight or stay longer in neonatal units, are at increased risk of infection. Rotavirus, especially in its new strains can cause severe diarrhea and dehydration in newborns and sick. It has been shown that rotavirus infection is associated with necrotizing enterocolitis in preterm infants during the outbreak in the neonatal unit. It has been observed a significantly higher incidence of episodes of bradycardia and apnea two days before and two days after the diagnosis of rotavirus infection in newborns.

The most commonly afflicted regions of the gastrointestinal tract with NEC include terminal ileum, ileocolic region, and ascending colon. In study by the NEC with Rotavirus infection involved the descending colon and rectum. Sharma et al. in a study in a neonatal intensive care unit with 2444 admissions, 129 had NEC. Thirty eight were rotavirus positive. Their findings also suggest that severe NEC, as characterized by diffuse pneumatosis, bacteraemia, and severe thrombocytopenia, is indistinguishable from advanced NEC associated with other organisms. They came to the conclusion that the neonatal mortality and morbidity in the severe form of NEC is similar by rotavirus or bacterial pathogens.

The measures to decrease NEC y rotavirus infection include increased awareness of rotavirus season in the community and maternal milk feedings. The maternal milk feedings seem to benefit against rotavirus infection because mucin, lactadherin, and antirotaviral antibodies present inhibit rotavirus binding with epithelial cells.

Co-infection with Salmonella Species

Rotavirus and nontyphoid Salmonella (NTS) were the most common pathogens cause of hospitalization of acute gastroenteritis in children. The incidence of coinfection Rotavirus and Salmonella NTS reported by published studies is 0.48-7.4%. The prevalence is higher in male children. However, in terms of clinical severity scores, there were no differences between males and females, were significantly related to a higher frequency of longer duration of diarrhea, longer length to hospitalization, and higher clinical severity score in comparison with rotavirus infection.

A study by Hung et al. reported that 70% of patients that were coinfected with both presented vomiting in comparison with 40% of patients with NTS infection only. However Wei-Te Lee et al., in a retrospective study in 2,040 hospitalized children in Taiwan report this phenomenon did not present in their study, but confirms that the clinical severity of NTS infection is worse than of rotavirus infection. Positivity for fecal leukocytes and fecal pus cells were found more frequently in coinfected patients.

Septicemia Following Rotavirus Gastroenteritis

Septicemia after rotavirus gastroenteritis is a rare but dangerous entity. To date, there are a few authors have compiled case series of this pathology. The incidence rate of 0.32% in the literature. Although this complication is apparently strange, the lack of descriptions is probably because not thinking about it and failure to obtain blood cultures later in course of rotavirus gastroenteritis.

The typical course for cases of bacteraemia superinfection involves a second peak of high fever (either recrudescence of fever or new onset fever in previously afebrile infants) several days after admission for rotavirus gastroenteritis. Presentation of symptoms can appear from the third day of illness to over a week, and not present a markedly elevated leukocyte count or inflammatory markers. Blood cultures should be obtained and considered empiric antibiotic therapy.

Bacteraemia occurred more commonly in immunocompromised patients and in neonates and young infants. Moreover, secondary bacteraemia by organisms of the normal intestinal flora has only been documented in Shigella gastroenteritis.

In 2005, there were the first descriptions by Lowental et al., report 1 neonate and 3 infants with bacteraemia secondary Enterobacter cloacae and Klebsiella pneumoniae, both normal commensals of the human small intestine. Morever, Scheier et al. in 2013 did a review of cases of rotavirus gastroenteritis and superimposed bacterial sepsis in the English literature; their findings were 20 cases in children, the most of all male. The organism findings: K. pneumoniae, (4) E. cloacae(4) ESBL – producing E. Coli (2), P. aeruginosa (1), Acinetobacter (1) C. albicans (2), K. oxytoca (1) and Pantea agglomerans, K oxytoca (1), Streptococcus viridans (1). All of them had fever major 39, 5ºC and higher levels of leukocyte count and/or CRP. The 20 cases of bacterial superinfection following rotavirus infection were reported from only a handful of countries: Japan, Brazil, Israel, Spain, Turkey and Italy. Regional and /or ethnic variation may provide diversity in an intestinal bacterial milieu, with possible consequences on the predisposition of children to develop septicaemia from occult bacteraemia.

How septicemia develops from Rotavirus infection is not fully understood. In these cases, initial blood cultures were sterile. It is, therefore, conceivable that the mucosal damage during rotavirus infection may be sufficient to allow bacterial translocation, leading to secondary bacteraemia, notably in the vulnerable intestinal wall of young infants. In 18 of than 20 cases the age of the children ranged between several weeks and 18 months, with only two patients above 3 years of age. It is presumed that immaturity of the intestinal barrier predisposes young infants to bacterial translocation, and this age distribution appears to be a factor.

Kawasaki Disease

Kawasaki disease (KD) is a multisystemic vasculitis, manifested by several signs and symptoms: fever, rash, conjunctival injections, cervical lymphadenopathy, oral mucosal changes, and extremity changes. Primarily affected are children less 5 years of age, and is more common in males. KD is a cause of acquired heart disease in children, approximately 22% - 4% (untreated - treated patients) develop coronary artery dilatation and aneurysm.

The etiology of KD is unclear. The history viral infection is strongly suspected, and a genetic component is important because of the widely varying frequencies in different racial and ethnic groups. Coinfection Rotavirus and H1N1 influenza A has been reported with incomplete Kawasaki disease.

VAERS (Vaccine Adverse Event Reporting System) is a national post marketing spontaneous reporting system for vaccine adverse events, jointly operated by the FDA.

KD can occur in a temporal relationship with vaccination, but a casual association has not been established. A review of RotaTeq (rotavirus vaccine, live, oral, pentavalent Merck&Co) clinical trial data revealed higher, though not statistically significantly (1.47/100,000 person-years). Although the majority of KD cases after other vaccines had onset on days 0 to 1 post vaccination, the intervals for RotaTeq cases spread out between 0 and 54 days post vaccination, with most occurring 2-30 days.

Acute Pancreatitis

Hyperamylasemia is relatively frequent, and is associated with severe gastroenteritis. However, acute pancreatitis in the setting of acute gastroenteritis is a rare event.

Acute pancreatitis is less common in children than in adults, but in the past two decades the incidence in the pediatric age has increased significantly. A wide variety of infectous agents (viruses, bacteria, fungi and parasites) have been associated, but only few cases due to rotavirus infection have been described.

This pathology is defined as requiring 2 of the following conditions: abdominal pain, serum amylase and/or lipase values $\geq$ 3 times upper limits of normal, and imaging findings of acute pancreatitis.

There are a few publications that describing the association acute pancreatitis and Rotavirus infection. All cases occurred in children with a median age of 2 years (range: 1-10 years). Most of them were male. Symptoms of rotavirus infection preceded the diagnosis in a 90% (from 2 to 10 days) of pancreatitis. Abdominal pain was rare. Imaging techniques showed moderately enlarged edematous pancreas in 3 cases. None of the patients underwent surgery or was referred to an intensive care unit. In 5-10 days all patients recovered the normalization of pancreatic enzymes.

The pathogenic mechanisms subtending pancreatic damage during infectious gastroenteritis are not clear. Rotaviruses infect mature enterocytes of the small intestine and, by an unknown mechanism, escape the gastrointestinal tract and cause viremia. Histopathological changes due to rotavirus infection included acute inflammation of the portal tract and bile duct. Another hypothesis could be the obstruction of pancreatic fluid outflow though and edematous ampulla of Vater have led to pancreatitis.

Elevated Levels of Serum Transaminase

Aminotransferases are normally present in circulation at low levels. They are intracellular enzymes produced principally by hepatocytes, and their increase in serum is therefore indicative of liver cell injury. However, aspartate aminotransferase (AST) is also found in cardiac and skeletal muscles, the kidneys, brain, pancreas, and lungs, and in erythrocytes, in decreasing order of concentration. Additionally, alanine aminotransferase (ALT) is present in skeletal muscle and kidneys, but at low concentrations, and its increase in the circulation is more specific for liver damage than AST. Aminotransferase serum levels depend not only on the tissue of origin, but also on the enzyme half-life, which is longer for ALT than AST.

Rotavirus is one of the leading causes of acute gastroenteritis among children. While clinical complaints are generally intestinal including vomiting and diarrhea, there is evidence to suggest that disease outside the gastrointestinal tract occurs. This study examines the frequency of hepatic transaminase elevation in children with rotavirus gastroenteritis. Patients identified with rotavirus gastroenteritis by stool antigen testing between November 2005 and March 2006 had available serum analyzed for alanine aminotransferase (ALT), aspartate aminotransferase (AST), alkaline phosphatase, total bilirubin, direct bilirubin, and creatinine phoshosphokinase (CPK). Chart review was conducted to identify patients with possible liver injury unrelated to rotavirus. Among the 92 patients identified with rotavirus during the study period, 75 had serum specimens available for testing. Fifteen patients (20%) had elevated ALT and AST, including one patient with an increase in AST, ALT, alkaline phosphatase, and total and direct bilirubin. The mean ALT elevation was 56 IU/L (range, 44 to 114 IU/L), and the mean AST elevation was 80 IU/L (range, 57 to 126 IU/L). Fifty-three patients (71%) had an increase in AST alone, and three patients (4%) had an increase in AST and alkaline phosphatase. The mean AST values in these groups were 61 IU/L (range, 42 to 110 IU/L) and 79 IU/L (range, 59 to 96 IU/L), respectively. In conclusion, rotavirus commonly causes elevation of liver transaminases.

Akelma et al. studied a total de 644 children who presented with acute gastroenteritis were assessed. 272 patients were diagnosed de rotavirus positive acute gastroenteritis, their findings were 15.4% elevated ALT and 25.4% (69 children) elevated AST. While the group with rotavirus negative acute gastroenteritis in 370 children obtained 6.8% and 11.9% respectively. These higher levels of serum transaminase were found to significantly higher in the group positive. During the follow up the levels of ALT and AST were normalized in both groups. These authors showed a clearly significantly a liver influence in rotavirus infection.

Sudden Infant Death Syndrome Associated with Rotavirus Infection

Sudden infant death syndrome is the sudden death of an infant that is not predicted by medical history and remains unexplained after a thorough forensic autopsy and detailed death scene investigation.

In 1982, Yolken described 5 cases of deceased children by in which detected rotavirus in their stool specimens, over a period of 3 weeks. The cases described showed no symptoms of acute gastroenteritis but 4 of them were suffering if upper respiratory infection. No other apparent cause found in them.

Rotavirus and Crohn´s Disease

The etiology of Crohn´s disease (CD) is currently unknown. In a summary the current literature surrounding the association between viruses and CD, were identified VEB, CMV. But there was little evidence by association with others viruses like Rotavirus. None of them has been proven as a real and exclusively pathogenic factor.

Intussusception

Intussusception is the invagination of one segment of the intestine within a more distal segment. It is the most common cause of bowel obstruction in infants, occurring usually between 4 and 10 months of age. If the intussusception is not relieved, the vascular supply of the bowel may be compromised, resulting in intestinal ischemia and possibly perforation. Untreated intussusception may be fatal.

In 1999, an association was found between a tetravalent rhesus reassortant rotavirus vaccine (RotaShield) and intussusception in US infants prompting the manufacturer to withdraw the vaccine from the market. Because of this association, the rotavirus vaccine that is currently recommended by the World Health Organization [RotaTeq (RV5), Merck & Co] was evaluated in large safety trials which excluded a risk of intussusception similar to that found with RotaShield (1 excess case per 10,000 vaccinated infants). However, postlicensure studies in some high and middle income settings have identified a low level risk of 1–2 excess cases of intussusception per 100,000 infants after this vaccine.

Studies assess the role of wild-type rotavirus infection as a cause of intussusception have led to conflicting findings with several studies suggesting that a significant association is unlikely. The absence of any marked seasonal patterns in intussusception, particularly in settings of Europe, Oceania, and Central and South America where rotavirus disease is quite seasonal supports the contention that rotavirus is unlikely to be a prominent etiologic cause of natural intussusception. This has some implications for post licensure monitoring because attempts have previously been made to assess whether rotavirus vaccination would have a protective effect against intussusception protecting against wild-type rotavirus infection. Establishing whether vaccine confers protection against intussusception might be challenging if only a small etiologic fraction of naturally occurring intussusception is related to wild-type rotavirus infection.

References

Abe T, Kobayashi M, Araki K, Kodama H, Fujita Y, Shizonaki T. Infantile convulsions with mild gastroenteritis. *Brain Dev.* 2000;22: 301-306.

American Academy of Pediatrics. Rotavirus infections. In: Pickering LK, Baker CJ, Long SS, eds RedBook: 2009 Report of the Committee on Infectious Diseases. 28 th ed. Elk Grove Village, IL: American Academy of Pediatrics, 2009: 576-9.

Carbonero-Celis MJ, De Cueto M, Carbonero-Santaella A, Haro Gómez M. Incomplete Kawasaki disease concomitant with influenza A H1N1 virus and rotavirus coinfection. *Enferm. Infecc. Microbiol. Clin.* 2013 Feb; 31(2):125-6.

Castello AA, Argüelles MH, Masini M, Villegas PD, Ghiringhelli PD, Semorille L, Glickmann G. Charaterization of human group C rotavirus in Argentina. 2000. *J. Med. Virol*: 62: 199-207.

Chiappini E, Galli L, de Martino M. Viremia and clinical manifestations in children with rotavirus infection. *J. Infect. Dis.* 2006 May 1;193(9):1333

Day TG, Jackson C, Bryant PA. Cluster of neurological manifestations of rotavirus infection in children. *BMJ Case Rep.* 2012 Mar 20; 2012.

Fernández MA, Madruga M, Blanco B, Rufo M. Estado epileptic asociado a una gastroenteritis leve por rotavirus. *An Pediatr (Barc).*2008;69(3)263-6.

Fukuda S, Kishi K, Kenji Y, Sejima H, Yamaguchi S. Rotavirus-associated encephalopathy with a reversible splenial lesion. *Pediatr. Neurol.* 2009;40:131-3.

Huang TS, Lu XG, Li B, Chen Y, Wen JL, Hu Y, Chen L, Xiao YH, Zhang J, Liao JX. [Benign infantile convulsions with mild gastroenteritis: clinical analysis of 40 cases]. Zhongguo Dang Dai Er Ke Za Zhi. 2010 Jul;12(7): 533-5.

Isik U, Caliskan M. Reversible EEG changes during rotavirus gastroenteritis. *Brain Dev.*2008;30:73-76.

Kang B, Kim D, Hong Y, Son B, Kim D, Kwon Y. Comparision between febrile and afebrile seizures associated with mild rotavirus gastroenteritis. *Seizure.*2013;22:560-4.

Karabel M, Karabel D, Kara S, Halıcı Taş T, Türkay S. [A rare cause of afebrile convulsion: rotavirus gastroenteritis]. *Arch. Argent Pediatr.* 2013 Apr;111(2):e43-5

Kawano G, Oshige K, Syutou S, Koteda Y, Yokoyama T, Kim BG, et al. Benign infantile convulsions associated with mild gastroenteritis: A retrospective study of 39 cases including virological tests and efficacy of anticonvulsants. *Brain Dev.* 2007 Nov;29(10):617-22.

Komori H, Wada M, Eto M, Oki H, Aida K, Fujimoto T. Benign convulsions associated with mild gastroenteritis: a report of 10 recent cases detailing clinical varieties. *Brain Dev.*1995;17:334-7.

Kubota T, Suzuki T, Kitase Y, Kidokoro H, Miyajima Y, Ogawa A, Natsume J, Okumura A. Chronological diffusion-weighted imaging changes and mutism in the course of rotavirus-associated acute cerebellitis/ cerebellopathy concurrent with encephalitis/encephalophaty. *Brain Dev.* 2011;33:21-27.

Lan WT, Lee HC, Yeung CY, Jiang CB, Kao HA, Hung HY, Chiu NC. Concomitant rotavirus and Salmonella infections in children with acute diarrhea. *Pediatr. Neonatol.* 2009 Feb;50(1):8-12.

Lee EH, Chung S. A comparative study of febrile and afebrile seizures associated with mild gastroenteritis. *Brain Dev.*2013;35:636-640.

Lee WT, Lin PC, Lin LC, Chen HL, Yang RC. Salmonella/rotavirus coinfection in hospitalized children. *Kaohsiung J. Med. Sci.* 2012 Nov;28(11):595-600.

Li T, Hong S, Peng X, Cheng M, Jiang L. Benign infantile convulsions associated with mild gastroenteritis: An electro clinical study of 34 patients. *Seizure.*2014;23:16-19.

Lloyd MB, Lloyd JC, Gesteland PH, Bale JF. Rotavirus gastroenteritis and seizures in young children. *Pediatr. Neurol.*2010;42:404-408.

Marti I, Cilla G, Gomáriz M, Eizaguirre J, Pérez Yarza EG. Rotavirus y crisis convulsivas. Una asociación poco frecuente aunque bien definida. *An Pediatr (Barc).* 2010; 73(2):70-73.

Naing Z, Rayner B, Killikulangara A, Vunnam K, Leach S, McIver CJ, Scott GM, Craig ME, Lui K, Rawlinson WD. Prevalence of viruses in stool of premature neonates at a neonatal intensive care unit. *J. Paediatr. Child Health.* 2013 Mar;49(3):E221-6.

Okumura A, Tanabe T, Kato T, Hayakawa F, Watanabe K. A pilot study on lidocaine tape therapy for convulsions with mild gastroenteritis. *Brain Dev.* 2004 Dec;26(8):525-9.

Ortiz O, Giménez F. Convulsiones afebriles asociadas a Rotavirus. *An Pediatr (Barc).*2008;69(4):383-95.

Panozzo CA, Tate JE, Payne DC, Cortese MM, Patel M. Reduction in rotavirus after vaccine introduction. United States, 2000-2009. *Morbility and Mortality Weekly Report.* October 23, 2009/58(41): 1146-1149.

Parashar UD, Gibson EG, Bresee JS, Milleer MA, Glass RI. Global Illness and deaths caused by rotavirus disease in children. 2003. *Emerging Infectious Diseases*, 9: 565-572.

Parashar UD, Gibson CJ, Breese. Rotavirus and severe childhood diarrhea. *2006 Emerging Infectious Diseases.* 12: 304-306.

Plana M, Fernández A, Vallmanya T, López A, Goma AR. Convulsiones afebriles y gastroenteritis aguda: una asociación más frecuente de lo esperado. *An Pediatr (Barc).*2008;69(3):267-70.

Regueras L, Iglesias C, Rodríguez C, Fernández L, Jiménez A, Recio V. Asociación entre gastroenteritis aguda leve y convulsiones afebriles benignas. *Bol. Pediatr.* 2010;50:21-24.

Shiihara T, Watanabe M, Honma A, Kato M, Morita Y, Ichiyama T, et al. Rotavirus associated acute encephalitis/encephalopathy and concurrent cerebellitis: Report of two cases. *Brain Dev.* 2007;29:670-673.

Sugata K, Taniguchi K, Yui A, Miyake F, Suga S, Asano Y, et al. Analysis of rotavirus antigenemia and extraintestinal manifestations in children with rotavirus gastroenteritis. *Pediatrics*.2008;122(2):392-7.

Tai IC, Huang YC, Lien RI, Huang CG, Tsao KC, Lin TY. Clinical manifestations of a cluster of rotavirus infection in young infants hospitalized in neonatal care units. *J. Microbiol. Immunol. Infect.* 2012 Feb;45(1):15-21.

Takanashi J, Miyamoto T, Ando N, Kubota T, Oka M, Kato Z, Hamano S, Karabel M, Karabel D, Kara S, Halıcı Taş T, Türkay S. A rare cause of afebrile convulsion: rotavirus gastroenteritis. *Arch. Argent Pediatr.* 2013 Apr;111(2):e43-5.

Takanashi J, Miyamoto T, Ando N, Kubota T, Oka M, Kato Z, Hamano S, Hirabayashi S, Kikuchi M, Barkovich AJ. Clinical and radiological features of rotavirus cerebellitis. *AJNR Am. J. Neuroradiol.* 2010 Oct;31(9):1591-5.

Thompson MJ, Gowdie PJ, Kirkwood CD, Doherty RR, Fahey M. Rotavirus cerebellitis: new aspect to an Old Foe?. *Pediatr. Neurol.* 2012;46:48-50.

Uemura N, Okumura A, Negoro T, Watanabe K. Clinical features of benign convulsions with mild gastroenteritis. *Brain Dev.* 2002;24(8):745-9.

Verotti A, Nanni G, Agostinelli S, Parisi p, Capovilla G, Beccaria F, et al. Benign convulsions associated with mild gastroenteritis: A multicenter clinical study. *Epilepsy Res.* 2011;93(2-3):107-14.

In: Rotavirus Infections
Editor: Carissa D. Zeni
ISBN: 978-1-63321-442-2

Chapter 3

Vaccination against Rotaviruses

***V. Bostik*[1,*], *M. Salavec*[2], *R. Sleha*[1] *and P. Bostik*[1]**
[1]Faculty of Military Health Sciences, University of Defence, Hradec Kralove, Czech Republic
[2]Department of Dermatovenereology, Charles University Medical School and University Hospital, Hradec Kralove, Czech Republic

Abstract

It is estimated that rotaviruses cause approximately 125 million cases of gastroenteritis worldwide annually. More than half a million of these cases lead to death and a majority of these fatal cases occur in the developing world. Humans are the source of infection and the fecal-oral route is the predominant mode of transmission. The infection shows a seasonal pattern in those countries of the temperate climate, which have not introduced a general vaccination schedule yet, and the incidence in these countries peaks in winter months. This has not been proven in tropical countries.

Standard hygienic and preventive measures are not hundred percent effective. Due to the fact that 10 virus particles is the minimal infective dose in humans, the vaccination is the only measure that offers a full

* Corresponding author: V. Bostik, Faculty of Military Health Sciences, University of Defence, Trebesska 1575, 500 01 Hradec Kralove, Czech Republic. Tel: (420) 973 253 205. E-mail address: vbostik@pmfhk.cz (Vanda Bostik).

prevention of the transmission of rotavirus infections in human population.

Introduction

Disorders manifesting as an acute gastroenteritis are the leading cause of morbidity and mortality in children in the age up to five years according to the WHO (World Health Organization) and CDC (Centres for Disease Control and Prevention) surveys. The incidence peak was persistently recorded in infants of 7 – 12 months of age [1, 2]. Such disorders rank at the top place of morbidity and mortality in many developing countries. Over seven hundred million cases of diseases associated with diarrhoea are reported every year in Africa, Asia and Latin America. Two to 3 million of these diseases in children annually are estimated to have a fatal outcome. Such data correspond to 6.600 – 9.000 deaths in children daily [3]. In the poorest population groups in Peru and Brasil children younger than two years suffer from diarrhoea more than ten times annually. In Costa Rica, a country with relatively good standards of living, the frequency of diarrhoea disease in children up to one year of age is 0.7 per annum [4, 5, 6].

Disorders manifesting as diarrhoea are caused by a number of agents including bacteria (*Vibrio cholerae, Shigella dysenteriae, Salmonella typhi, Campylobacter, Clostridium difficile, Escherichia coli, Listeria monocytogenes, Salmonella enteritidis*), parasites (*Cryptosporidium parvum, Giardiasis lambda*) and viruses (rotaviruses, noroviruses, adenoviruses, astroviruses).

It is very difficult to determine the exact causative agents of such disorders due to insufficient laboratory diagnostics, particularly in developing countries [3, 7, 8].

Epidemiology of Rotaviruses

It has been known for some time that rotaviruses (family *Reoviridae* including the genus *Rotavirus* and *Coltivirus*) represent the most common cause of acute gastroenteritis associated with dehydration in infants and children in both developing and countries [9, 10]. It is estimated that rotaviruses are the causative agents in more than 125 million of gastroenteritis cases in children, resulting in 418.000-520.000 deaths. Eighty five percent of these cases happen in developing countries [3].

In the USA, almost every unvaccinated child up to one year of age experiences rotavirus infection with symptomatic gastroenteritis. During the ongoing rotavirus vaccination campaign in the USA, 73% of children younger than 1 year of age, 64% of children older than 1 year of age and 8% of children in the age of 2-4 years were vaccinated at least by 1 dose by the end of 2008. Data from 2007-2008 demonstrated a 75% decrease in hospitalization due to vaccination compared to the pre-vaccination period. In 2008-2009 the decrease of incidence of 60% was recorded [3, 11, 12].

In the Czech Republic underreporting of rotavirus gastroenteritis has been expected on behalf of *Salmonella* and *Campylobacter* infections. In the "Epidat" system, some 2800 cases of viral diarrhoea were recorded between 2006-2009 with the majority of reports in hospitalized patients. It is estimated that 1600 cases of the total were caused by rotavirus infection, particularly in children up to 3 years of age. The realistic estimation leads to some 20.000 rotavirus infection cases in the Czech Republic annually [13, 14, 15].

Number of published papers refer to a seasonal character of rotavirus infections in countries of temperate climate, while such seasonal pattern is absent in tropical countries.

Winter months – December to March on North Hemisphere and June to September on the South Hemisphere – are considered as a period of the highest incidence of rotavirus infections in countries of temperate climate. On the contrary, non-seasonal character in tropical countries has been attributed to different climatic conditions such as local air circulation, pressure zone, or degree of variability of sunlight in each particular zone throughout the year.

In a summary, local climatic factors may influence seasonal prevalence of rotavirus infections in different areas of the world [18].

Rotaviruses are not the only viruses where such seasonal occurrence could be observed. Herpetic virus varicella-zoster (VZV) displays similar manner of seasonal variation in countries with temperate climate in contrast to all-season prevalence in tropical countries [19].

Molecular Biology of Rotavirus

Rotavirus is a nonenveloped, double-stranded, RNA virus, discovered and described in 1973.

The size of rotavirus virion is 65 -75 nm in average. Virus is composed of the icosahedral nucleus and two-layer capsid [20]. Nucleus is formed by double-stranded RNA containing 11 segments, which encode 6 structural (VP) and 6 non-structural proteins (NSP) [21].

Rotavirus is the only mammalian virus with described double-stranded RNA organized into segments. The sizes of the individual segments are different, e.g., segment 11 contains 667 pair base-pairs while segment 1 contains 3 302 bp. The total nucleic RNA length is about 18 500 bp depending on the particular viral strain. It is interesting that rotavirus sequences are rich in A-T bases (58-67%). Viral nucleus is composed of VP1, VP2 and VP3 proteins, which are coded for by genes 1, 2 and 3. All 11 segments code for both viral structural and non-structural proteins, but their function has been identified in only about 50% [22, 23, 24, 25, 26].

The outer layer contains two proteins, VP4 (P protein) and VP7 (G protein). VP7 is a glycoprotein coded by genes 7, 8 or 9. VP4 is a glycoprotein coded by gene 4. About 90% of the capsid surface is composed of VP7 with 132 channels perforating virion and extending to the nucleus [27]. VP4 influences both rotavirus virulence and its binding to specific receptors [28]. These surface proteins induce independently production of neutralizing antibodies in host and, as such, play a fundamental role in rotavirus vaccine design [28]. About 20 P and G serotypes of the virus can be distinguished based on antigenic structure.

The other important protein is VP6 coded for by gene 6, which is localized in the internal layer of the capsid and makes up about 51% of the virus structure. [29].

According to antigenic structure of the internal layer of the capsid, rotaviruses are classified into serologic groups marked A – L [30]. The group A includes serologic types G1, G2, G3, G4 and G9. These serologic types are associated with geographical and seasonal prevalence, but no relationship to the severity of the clinical course has been identified [30, 31].

Based on molecular genetic analyses at least 19 G genotypes have been detected in humans and animals representing 14 serologic types and further 27 P genotypes represent additional 18 serologic types [32, 33]. Combination of G and P types creates basis for so-called binomic standardization used to identify particular rotavirus strains. Theoretically, this allows for more than 110 different combinations of G and P types.

Nevertheless, G serologic types G1-G4 and G9 and P genotypes P4 and P8 are most frequent worldwide and are responsible for 90% of infections in developed countries and for 68% of infections in South America and in Asia.

Globally, the predominant genotype is P [8]-G1, followed by P [8]–G3, P [4] – G2 and P [8]–G4 [34, 35]. The G9 genotype was determined around the year 2000 for the first time and is regarded as predominant in some areas in Europe, Thailand and in some parts of Eastern Asia. Less common serotypes are P [6]-G8 in Africa, P [8] – G5 in Brasilia and P [11] –G10 and P [6] – G12 in India [36, 37].

The predominant fraction of human rotavirus isolates belong to the group A and therefore vaccines are primarily prepared to target this group. As a matter of fact, only this group includes viruses responsible for severe gastroenteritis with possible dehydration of epidemiologic significance [38]. Infections caused by the B group of rotaviruses were identified in China and are characterized by diarrhoeal disorders mainly in adult patients [39]. The group C rotavirus infections are extremely rare in children in different countries worldwide and are more characteristic for animals, especially pigs [40]. The remaining rotavirus groups D-G have not been detected in human population and are found most commonly in primates, cattle, horses, pigs and in sheep [40].

Molecular genetic studies based on comparisons of individual genomic segments proved an existence of genetic shift (Re-assortment) and drift mechanisms analogous to the influenza virus type A. Although the serologic types of animal rotaviruses are different from the strains with the highest prevalence in humans, there is a high homology between the individual animal and human strains. It is assumed that such similarity originated due to the re-assortment of one or more animal rotavirus genes into human rotavirus genome during *in vivo* infections [40].

Ways of Transmission, Infection Sources, Risk Groups

The most common way of transmission is the faecal-oral route, especially by hand contamination. Transmission through the respiratory route by air drops has been speculated, but it is still regarded as undemonstrated hypothesis. However, it seems plausible to include respiratory symptoms into clinical presentation of rotavirus infections [41].

Health-care staff, pediatricians, geriatric units, rest home and day-care service staff, as well as infant schools and day nurseries belong to risk groups.

Immunocompromised patients including HIV/AIDS patients belong to risk groups as well [42].

Rotaviruses are classified as common hospital nosocomial pathogens at pediatric departments. About 5 – 30% of pediatric patients develop diarrhoea during hospitalization [41]. The frequent source of infection is contaminated food – particularly food not treated by heat, such as vegetable salads, insufficiently rinsed fruit, contaminated water and ice [42].

Depending on the type of material, rotaviruses survive on various surfaces for a different time. Studies testing survival times of virulent viruses on toys with different surface types demonstrated an ability of the virus to survive up to several days on plastic, rubber, metal or wooden material, whereas virus survival only in hours was demonstrated on skin of hands [43, 44, 45].

It was verified experimentally that the best antiseptic agent to combat rotavirus is alcohol (99% efficacy) compared only to 72-84% efficacy when ordinary soap and water were used, which is one of the reasons supporting vaccination as the optimal way to combat rotavirus infection. As mentioned above, only 10 virions represent a sufficient infection dose in a child... In a frozen form (-60 C), rotavirus can survive several years, while the temperature of 56 C inactivates rotavirus in 30 minutes. UV rays damage viral particles in several minutes [46, 47].

Virus is stable at pH 3.5-10 and its passage through the stomach acid barrier is therefore improved, if the mucosal pH is increased. Under normal circumstances with pH 2 in stomach, virus survives maximally one minute, but the stomach pH in infants is about 3, 2 and so such environment is more permissive for the passage of the virulent virus into the gastrointestinal tract.

Clinical Course of Rotavirus Infection

Rotavirus infection is usually restricted to gut mucosa. Rotavirus adheres to mature epithelial cells in the tips of villi in upper 2/3 of small intestine (most commonly in duodenum and in proximal part of jejunum) by viral VP4 protein and replicates there massively during 1-2 days [15, 33, 41]. Mature viral particles are released due to the disintegration of epithelial cells and infect other cells. New virions mature and are released in 10-12 hour-cycles [47]. The gut injury caused by viruses leads to a substantial decrease of salt and water absorption. Dyspepsia and malabsorption occur due to the destruction of gut cells (enterocytes), resulting in osmotic diarrhoea, vomiting and dehydration.

The diseases course is approximately 5-7 days. Typical symptoms include vomiting, fever, abdominal pain and profuse nonhemorrhagical diarrhoea. The essential problem is dehydration in about 2% of cases. If no sufficient rehydration management is available, shock, electrolyte dysbalance and subsequently death could occur. Vomiting and fever (fever above 39 C in about 1/3 of patients) are typical in first two to three days of the disease, whereas diarrhea persists usually for 5-8 days [48]. The immunity acquired after the infection is not complete and multiple recurrences could occur with milder disease compared to first presentation. Breast-feeding does not provide protection against rotavirus infection, but it is assumed that the manifestations of the disease are milder in breastfed infants [49, 50, 51]. The infection in adults can occur, but they are more often asymptomatic based on longitudinal studies in several countries [52, 53].

Rotavirus Vaccine Development

The principal strategy for efficient rotavirus vaccine is to obtain vaccine inducing life-long immunity to life-threatening diarrhoeal disorders resulting in dehydration. The first candidate vaccines were derived from monovalent bovine or monkey (*Rhesus macaque*) rotavirus strains. Trials with such vaccines applied in dose scheme demonstrated safety of orally administrated vaccine, inducing immunity against rotavirus infections in children. However, the efficacy of such vaccines was not consistent. In spite of fact that vaccines induced a heterotypic antibody response, an opinion prevailed to develop a multivalent vaccine with greater confidence to induce specific immunity against all major pathogenic strains of rotaviruses [53]. It should be noted, however, that the 2 currently licensed living oral vaccines available, monovalent and pentavalent, demonstrate a comparable level of safety and efficacy [54, 55].

The first rotavirus vaccines were based on Edward Jenner´s postulate, dated more than 200 years ago: a related living attenuated pathogen of non-human origin could act as an immunogen when inserted into human organism [56]. Therefore the first candidate vaccines contained attenuated bovine rotavirus strain NCDV (Nebraska calf diarrhoea virus) [56]. During the last decade of the 20th century number of other candidate vaccines using bovine or monkey strains were successively developed and tested (MMV 18006 strain, virus from young *rhesus macaque*).

In 1998, RRV-TV RotaShield vaccine (Wyeth Laboratories, Inc., Marietta, Pennsylvania, USA) was licensed by the FDA (Food and Drug Administration, USA). This vaccine was indicated for pediatric use in the USA and administered orally. The vaccine was based on the reassortment of the genetic material of concurrent infections of human and monkey rotavirus strains. The application was performed in three doses – in 2, 4 and 6 months of life. During the subsequent 11 months approximately 1.5 million doses were administered in about 900,000 children [57]. In July 1999, the vaccine was withdrawn from the market due to the evaluation of the VAERS (Vaccine Adverse Event Reporting System), which reported 15 cases of intussusception (invagination of a part of the intestine into the following segment) in the vaccinated children group [57, 58]. In October 1999, some 114 cases of intussusception in the VAERS were reported and 99 cases were definitely confirmed. Out of these 99 cases, 49 appeared following the first vaccine dose, 10 case following the second one and only 1 case after the third dose. One case in 5-months old infant resulted in death.

Further vaccine development focused on testing of vaccines based on human rotavirus strains. The first such isolate was obtained from a day-nursery infant from Venezuela with asymptomatic rotavirus infection. Theory was based on studies from Australia, Sweden, UK and Venezuela demonstrating natural attenuation of human rotavirus strains in children [59]. The virus in this first tested vaccine of human origin, called M 37, was in tissue culture 29 times before use. Other isolates were tested at the same time, but efficacy studies did not show satisfactory results.

Current Rotavirus Vaccines

Two vaccines - RotaTeq (Merck, Sharp & Dohme) and Rotarix (GSK) are currently available. Both vaccines are highly immunogenic and protective [61]. RotaTeq is a live, attenuated, pentavalent bovine-human reassortant rotavirus vaccine administered orally. Four of these five rotaviruses express capsid proteins serotypes G1, G2, G3 or G4 from the human rotavirus parent strain. The fifth reassortant virus expresses the P1A protein from the human rotavirus parent strain and the outer capsid protein VP7 (serotype G6) from the bovine rotavirus parent strain. The individual strains are prepared separately and propagated in Vero cells. Bovine strains are attenuated „naturally", because they replicate poorly in human body. Vaccine is administered since six weeks of age in three doses with at least four weeks interval. Vaccination should be finished until twenty, maximally twenty-two weeks of age [62].

Rotarix is a human, monovalent, live attenuated oral rotavirus vaccine containing strain RIX4414 of the most frequent serotype G1P, also propagated in Vero cells. Vaccine is administered after six weeks the age in two doses with at least four weeks interval. Vaccination should be finished until twenty-four weeks of age [63].

No recommendations on food, drink and breast feeding restrictions both before and following vaccination are indicated. Vaccines could not interchange during the course of vaccination. Both vaccines are well tolerated but due to prior problems with RothaShield vaccine, new vaccines are contraindicated in infants with a history of intussusception or with congenital malformation of the gastrointestinal tract [64].

The WHO has recommended an implementation of rotavirus vaccination into national vaccination programmes, stressing out the significance of rotavirus vaccination in developing countries, where high mortality rates is common. The WHO considers implementation of the vaccination as the most important measure in countries, where mortality rate in children less than five years of age is 10% and more. The WHO does not prefer either vaccine and recommends first administration in the age of 6-15 weeks concluding the vaccination until the age of 32 weeks.

Routine vaccinations are performed in 14 countries on American and European continents at present. Vaccine was also implemented in Guyana, Honduras, Nicaragua and Bolivia. North Sudan is the first country of African continent, which opened a vaccination campaign in summer of 2011. The GAVI (Global Alliance for Vaccines and Immunizations) foundation proposes in cooperation with the WHO a vaccination campaign enrolling 50 million children from 40 poorest world countries and anticipates concluding the vaccination before the end of 2015 [65].

In conclusion it could be summarized that a positive impact of rotavirus vaccination has been proven and its implementation will have great impact on the morbidity and mortality of young children worldwide.

References

[1] Meloni A, Locci D, Frau G. Epidemiology and prevention of rotavirus infection; an underestimated issue? *J. Matern. Fetal. Neonatal. Med.* 2011; Suppl 2: 48-51.

[2] Moore SR, Lima AA, Guerrant RL. Infection: Preventing 5 million child death from diarrhoea in the next 5 years. *Nat. Rev. Gastroenterol. Hepatol.* 2011; 8: 363-4.

[3] Rotavirus surveillance worldwide-2009. *Wkly Epidemiol. Rec.* 2011; 86: 174-6.

[4] Black RE, Lopez de Romana G, Brown KH et al. Incidence and etiology of infantile diarrhoea and major routes of transmission in Huascar, Peru. *Am. J. Epidemiol.* 1989; 129:785-99.

[5] Schorling JB, Wanke CA, Schorling SK et al. A prospective study of persistent diarrhoea among children in urban Brazilian slums. Patterns of occurrence and etiologic agents. *Am. J. Epidemiol.* 1990; 132:144-56.

[6] Simhon A, Mata L, Vives M et al. Low endemicity and low pathogenicity of rotaviruses among rural children in Costa Rica. *J. Infect. Dis.* 1985; 152:1134-42.

[7] Latipov R, Utegenova E, Kuatbayeva K. et al. Epidemiology and burden of rotavirus disease in Central Asia. *Int. J. Infect. Dis.* 2011; 15: e464-9.

[8] Fischer Walker CL, Black RE. Rotavirus vaccine and diarrhoea mortality: quantifying regional variation in effect size. *BMC Public Health.* 2011; Suppl#:S16.

[9] Cook SM, Glass RI, LeBaron CW. Global seasonality of rotavirus infections. *Bull. World Health Organ.* 1990; 68:171-7.

[10] Kapikian AZ. Overview of viral gastroenteritis. *Arch. Virol. Suppl.* 1996; 12:7-19.

[11] Glass RI, Patel M, Parashar U. Lessons from the US rotavirus vaccination program. *JAMA*.2011; 306:1701-2.

[12] Cortes JE, Curns AT, Tate JE et al. Rotavirus vaccine and health care utilization for diarrhoea in US children. *N. Engl. J. Med.* 2011; 365: 1108-17.

[13] Pazdiora P, Taborska J, Svecova M. Long-term follow-up of nosocomial rotavirus infections at the Infectious Diseases Clinic (1987-19940. *EMI* 1996; 45:95-100.

[14] Pazdiora P, Svecova M. Serologic overview of rotavirus antibodies in children under 2 years of age. *EMI*.1997; 46:34-5.

[15] Pazdiora P, Benes C. Diagnosis and notification of rotavirus infection in the Czech Republic. *EMI.* 2000; 49:16-8.

[16] Bhowmick K, Kang G, Bose A et al. retrospective surveillance for intussusceptions in children aged less than 5 years in a South Indian territorium. *J. Health Popul. Nutr.* 2009; 27:660-5.

[17] Atchison C, Lopman B, Edmunds WJ. Modeling the seasonality of rotavirus disease and the impact of vaccination in England and Wales. *Vaccine*. 2010; 19:3118-26.

[18] Levy K, Hubbard AE, Eisenberg JN. Seasonality of rotavirus disease in the tropics: a systematic review and meta-analysis. *Int. J. Epidemiol.* 2009; 38:1487-96.

[19] Enskhsaikhan D, Loparev VN, Bostik V, et al. Genotyping of VZV strains isolated in Mongolia. *Vopr. Virusol.* 2010; 55:40-3.

[20] Ruiz MC, Leon T, Diaz Y et al. Molecular biology of rotavirus entry and replication. *Scientific World J.* 2009; 9:1476-97.

[21] da Silva MF, Tort LF, Gomez MM et al. Phylogenetic analysis of VP1, VP2, and VP3 gene segments of genotype G group A rotavirus strains. *Virus Res*. 2011; 160:381-8.

[22] Donker NC, Foley M, Tamvakis DC et al. Identification of an antibody-binding epitope on the rotavirus A non-structural protein NSP2. *J. Gen. Virol.* 2011; 92:2374-82.

[23] Akita F, Miyazaki N, Hibino H et al. Viroplasm matrix protein Pns9 from rice gall dwarf virus forms an octameric cylindrical structure. *J. Gen. Virol.* 2011; 92:2214-21.

[24] Top KA, Esquilin JM, Yen C et al. Detection of mutations in antigenic regions of rotavirus viral proteins 4 and 7. *Pediatric Infect. Dis.* 2011; 30:630.

[25] McDonald SM, Patton JT. Rotavirus VP2 core shell regions critical for viral polymerase activation. *J. Virol.* 2011; 85:3095-105.

[26] Ghosh S, Paul SK, Hossain MA et al. Full genomic analyses of two human G2P [4] rotavirus strains detected in 2005. *J. Gen. Virol.* 2011; 92:1222-7.

[27] McDonald SM, Patton JT. Assortment and packing of the segmented rotavirus genome. *Trends Microbiol.* 2011; 19:136-44.

[28] Ghosh S, Adachi N, gather Z et al. Whole genome analysis reveals the complex evolutionary dynamics of Kenyan G2P human rotavirus. *J. Gen. Virol.* 2011; 92:2201-8.

[29] Zhou H, Guo L, Wang M et al. prime immunization with rotavirus VLP 2/6 followed by boosting with an adenovirus expressing VP6. *Virol. J.* 2011; 5:8-3.

[30] Kirkwood CD. Genetic and antigenic diversity of human rotaviruses: potential impact on vaccination programs. *J. Infect. Dis.* 2011; 1,S43-8.

[31] Steele AD, Page N, de Beer M et al. Antigenic and molecular characterization of unusual rotavirus strains in Burkina faso in 1999. *J. Infect. Dis.* 2010; 202, S225-30.
[32] O Ryan M. The ever-changing landscape of rotavirus serotypes. *Pediatr. Infect. Dis. J.* 2009; 28:S60-2.
[33] Velazquez FR. Protective effects of natural rotavirus infection. *Pediatr. Infect. Dis.* 2009; 28:S54-6.
[34] Antunes H, Afonso A, Itrurriza M et al. G2P the most prevalent rotavirus genotype in 2007 winter season. *J. Clin. Virol.* 2009; 45:76-8.
[35] Karsten C, Baumgarte S, friedrich AW et al. Incidence and risk factors for community-acquired acute gastroenteritis in north-west Germany in 2004. *Eur. J. Clin. Micribiol. Infect. Dis.*2009; 28:935-43.
[36] Kiulia NM, Nyaundi JK, Peenze I et al. Rotavirus infection among HIV-infecetd children in Nairobi, Kenya. *J. Trop. Pediatr.* 2009; 55:318-23.
[37] Kamel AH, Ali MA, ElNady HG et al. Predominance and circulation of enteric viruses in the region of Greater Cairo, Egypt. *J. Clin. Microbiol.* 2009; 47:1037-45.
[38] Ushijima H, Ishida S. Rotavirus vaccine. *Nihon. Rinsho.* 2008; 66:1977-83.
[39] Jin Y, Chneg WX, Yang XM et al. Viral agents associated with acute gastroenteritis in children hospitalized with diarrhea in China. *J. Clin. Virol.* 2009; 44:238-41.
[40] Midgley SE, Banyai K, Buesa J et al. Diversity and zoonotic potential of rotaviruses in swine and cattle across Europe. *Vet. Microbiol.* 2012; 156:238-45.
[41] Taborska J, Pazdiora P. Rotaviruses – the most often problem in children's dirrhea. *Pediatry in practise.* 2005; 3:135-9.
[42] Cunningham, AL, Grohman GS, Harkness J et al. Gastrointestinal viral infections in homosexual men who were symptomatic and seropositive. *J. Infect. Dis.* 1988; 158:386-91.
[43] Goodgame RW. Viral causes of diarrhea. *Gastroenterol. Clin. North Am.* 2001; 30:779-95.
[44] Glass RI, Bresee J, Jiang B et al. Gastroenteritis viruses: an overview. *Novartis. Found Symp.* 2001; 238:5-19.
[45] Oliverira CS, Linhares AC.Rotavirus: clinical features and prevention. *J Pediatr.* 199; 75:S91-102.
[46] Ojeh CK, Cusak TM, Yolken RH. Evaluation of the effects of disinfectants on rotavirus RNA and infectivity by the polymerase chain recation methods. *Mol. Cell Probes.* 1995; 9:341-6.

[47] Li D, Gu AZ, He M et al. UC inactivation and resistance of rotavirus evaluated by integrated cell culture and real time PCR. *Water Res*. 2009; 43: 3261-9.

[48] Grenberg HB, Estes MK. Rotaviruses: from pathogenesis to vaccination. *Gastroenterology*. 2009; 1939-51.

[49] Desselberger U, Manktelow E, li W et al. Rotaviruses and rotavirus vaccines. *Br. Med. Bull.* 2009; 90:37-51.

[50] Parashar UD, Gibson CJ, Bresse JS et al. Rotavirus and severe childhood diarrhea. *Emerg. Infect. Dis.* 2006; 12:304-6.

[51] Forster J, Guarino A, Parez N et al. Hospital based surveillance to estimate the burden of rotavirus gastroenteritis among European children younger than 5 years of age. *Pediatrics*. 2009; 123:393-400.

[52] Phioips G, Lopman B, Rodrigues LC et al. Asymptomatic rotavirus infections in England: prevalence, characteristics, and risk factors. *Am. J. Epidemiol.* 2010; 171:1023-30.

[53] Eckardt AJ, Baumgart DC. Viral gastroenteritis in adults. *Recent Pat. Antiinfect. Drug Discov*. 2011; 6:54-63.

[54] Gray J. Rotavirus vaccines: safety, efficacy and public health impact. *J. Intern. Med.* 2011; 270:206-14.

[55] Tate JE, Parashar UD. Monitoring impact and effectiveness of rotavirus vaccination. *Expert. Rev. Vaccines.* 2011; 10:1123-5.

[56] Kawamura N. Rotavirus vaccine. *Nihon Rinsho*. 2011; 69:1609-15.

[57] Dennehy PH. Rotavirus vaccine: an overview. *Clin. Microbiol. Rev*. 2008. 21; 198-208.

[58] Matson DO. Rota Shield: the ill fated rhesus human reassortant rotavirus vaccine. *Pediatr. Ann.* 2006; 35:54-61.

[59] Ward RL, MvNeal MM, Steele AD. Why does the world need another rotavirus vaccine? *Ther. Clin. Risk Manag*. 2008; 4:49-63.

[60] Glass RI, Bressee JS, Turcios R et al. Rotavirus vaccine: targeting the developing world. *J. Infect. Dis.* 2005; 192:S160-6.

[61] Vesikari T., Giaguinto C., Huppertz HI. Clinical trials of rotavirus vaccine in Europe. *Pediatr. Infect. Dis*. 2006; 25:S42-7.

[62] ElKhoury AC, Mast TC, Ciarlet M et al. projecting the effectiveness of RotaTeq against rotavirus-related hospitalizations in Brazil. *Mem. Inst. Oswaldo Cruz*. 2011; 106:541-5.

[63] Plosker GL. Rotavrius vaccine RIX4414. *Pharmacoeconomics*. 2011; 29: 439-54.

[64] Lob Levyt J. Contribution of the GAVI Alliance to improving health and reducing poverty. *Philos. Trans. R Soc. Lond B Biol. Sci.* 2011, 12; 2473-7.

[65] Nossai GJ. Vaccines and future global health needs. *Philos. Trans. R Soc. Lond B Biol. Sci.* 2011;366:2833-40.

In: Rotavirus Infections
Editor: Carissa D. Zeni

ISBN: 978-1-63321-442-2

Chapter 4

Passive Immunity Strategies to Control Rotavirus Diarrhea in Neonatal Calves

Celina G. Vega and Viviana Parreño [*]
Instituto de Virologia, CICV y A, INTA, Castelar, Argentina

Abstract

The passive transfer of maternal immunity provides essential protection in the newborns. It is well known that the neonatal immune system of mammals and birds is fully competent to mount a primary immune response against infection, developing optimal levels of humoral and cell-mediated immunity. However, it is also known that after birth, newborns are exposed to a great variety of antigens for the first time. The initiation of several primary immune responses to those antigens, which in many cases cause mixed infections and complications, would not be quick or strong enough to overwhelm pathogen replication. Therefore, unless adequate maternal immunologic assistance is provided, neonates have an increased probability of dying after infection with common pathogens. Maternal immunologic assistance thus can provide a critical (though temporary) aid to survival for neonates. The evolutionary process developed effective mechanisms for the passive transfer of both systemic and mucosal immunity from the mother to her offspring. Taking

[*] Corresponding author: Email: vega.celina@inta.gob.ar, parreno.viviana@inta.gob.ar.

advantage of this natural process, vaccination of the dams has become a well-established practice among veterinary practitioners to prevent neonatal diseases. Dam vaccination increases the levels of passive maternal antibodies transferred from the mother via colostrum and milk intake. This strategy of passive systemic immunity had been applied with optimal results, especially for systemic infections. For enteric infections such as rotavirus caused diarrhea, dam vaccination had been the tool selected to reduce the severity of the disease and morbidity rates in cattle and horses.

A complementary or alternative strategy to prevent enteric diseases has been the oral administration of colostrum replacers and immune milk supplemented with protective levels of specific antibodies. Different sources of antibodies, i.e., oral administration of hyper immune plasma; fluid or powdered bovine immune colostrum, fluid or powdered chicken egg yolk IgY enriched in rotavirus-specific antibodies, have been explored and represents effective immunotherapies to prevent rotavirus diarrhea.

Passive immunity has been documented to often interfere with newborn active immune responses to natural infections and vaccination. In the recent years, the transference of immune cells and other biomolecules with immunomodulatory properties from the mother to their offspring had been described shedding light on the mechanism behind this interference. New adjuvants, antigen delivery systems and rationale vaccines designs to overwhelm or take advantage of the properties of these passive maternal biomolecules and cells transferred to the newborns are under development. This review will address current knowledge regarding the mechanism behind the protective and immunomodulatory effect of passive immunity strategies to prevent rotavirus diarrhea in the veterinary field.

Introduction

Development of the Neonatal Immune System

The immune system protects the host against pathogenic organisms and highly complex pathways of recognition, response, elimination and memory have evolved in order to fulfill this role. A breakdown in these pathways or their inefficient operation can lead to increased susceptibility to, and increased morbidity and mortality as a result of, infectious disease. The immune system also acts to ensure tolerance to 'self', to food and other environmental components, and to commensal bacteria. A breakdown in the tolerogenic pathways can also lead to so-called inflammatory diseases. However, both development and maintenance of tolerance are lifelong processes which start very early in life, even prenatally (Barrington & Parish, 2001; Battersby & Gibbons, 2013).

The passive transfer of maternal immunity provides essential protection in newborns. Although the neonatal immune system of mammals and birds is fully competent to develop primary immune responses against infection, newborn animals suddenly encounter a hostile microbial environment where they need to discriminate dietary antigens from pathogens. This is critical not only during this early stage of life but also because the response patterns "learned" during this period persist into adult life (Holt & Jones, 2000). The antigenic inexperience and the prevalence of suppression factors during fetal life are responsible for the "antigenic immaturity" of the immune system in newborns. Because it requires time and energy to develop a primary immune response, this occurs under the "protective umbrella" of passive maternal antibodies and immune cells transferred from the mother to the offspring by different mechanisms according to the species (Baintner, 2007).

After birth, newborns are exposed to a great variety of antigens for the first time. Acquisition of commensal microbiota after birth promotes maturation and regulation of the neonatal immune system and establishment of gut homeostasis (Chatthaa et al., 2014). Two important periods of maximum exposure to novel antigens occur in the young animal: immediately after birth and at weaning. In both cases, the antigenic composition of the intestinal contents can shift suddenly, as a result of a novel diet and of colonization by novel strains and species of bacteria (Bailey et al., 2007). The initiation of several primary immune responses to those antigens, which in many opportunities cause mixed infections and complications, may not be quick or strong enough to overwhelm pathogen replication. Therefore, unless adequate maternal immunologic assistance is provided, neonates have an increased probability of dying after infection with common pathogens.

Interestingly, most of this immunological bond between the mother and her newborn begins in the gut mucosa. In fact, the intestine is the largest immune organ in the body, and as such is the location for the majority of lymphocytes and other immune effector cells. The intestine is exposed to vast quantities of dietary and microbial antigens, and is the most common portal of entry for pathogens, some of which are potentially lethal. The development of normal immune function of the intestine is vital for survival, and is dependent on appropriate antigen exposure and processing, and also an intact intestinal barrier (Kelly & Coutts, 2000). Then, the mucosal immune system fulfils the primary function of defense against potential pathogens that may enter across vulnerable surface epithelia. as has been mentioned, the intestinal immune system discriminates between pathogen-associated and 'harmless' antigens, expressing active responses against the former and tolerance to the latter (Bailey et al., 2007).

Immediately after birth, newborns suck a dietary and immunologically rich secretion from their mothers: the colostrum. Maternal colostrum and milk, in addition to providing the newborn with nutrition, also confer immunological advantages and protect against gastrointestinal and respiratory diseases. Colostrum and milk not only confer passive protection, they have the ability to directly stimulate immune function. The precise pathways involved are not completely clear but the protective advantages conferred to the sucking infant can be grouped into four main categories comprising maturational, immuno-modulatory, anti-inflammatory and anti-microbial effects (Kelly & Coutts, 2000). The mechanisms of enhancing disease resistance are thought to be passive, involving a direct supply of anti-microbial factors, and active, by promoting the development of specific immune function. A tolerance response to dietary and non-invasive antigens is generally induced in the gut. The education of the immune system in early life is thought to be critical in minimizing the occurrence of immune-based disorders. During this phase of development, maternal colostrum and milk provide signals to the immune system that generate appropriate response and memory (Kelly & Coutts, 2000).

Colostrum Intake and Neonatal Fc Receptor

Maternal immunologic assistance provides a critical (though temporary) aid to survival for neonates. Through the evolutionary process, effective mechanisms have been developed to assure the passive transfer of both systemic and mucosal immunity from the mother to her offspring. As previously mentioned, it should be realized that the induction of an immune response against non-harmful common environmental antigens, such as food antigens and particular commensals (bacteria), has to be inhibited lest it gives rise to undesirable, excessive, and destructive inflammatory and allergic reactions (M'Rabet, Vos, Boehm, & Garssen, 2008). Therefore, successful absorption of colostrum is essential for disease prevention and growth of healthy animals.

Immunomodulatory and antimicrobial factors including antibodies and a variety of cells are integral parts of colostrum (Bandrick, Ariza-Nieto, Baidoo, & Molitora, 2014; Chatthaa et al., 2014; Nguyen et al., 2007). Maternal immunoglobulins are concentrated from the mother´s blood into colostrum in the mammary gland via an Fc-receptor dependent mechanism (Hammer & Mossmann, 1978). Lymphocytes derived from the common mucosal immune system migrate to the mammary gland and can be found in colostrum (Nguyen et al., 2007; Salmon, Berri, Gerdts, & Meurens, 2009; Tuboly & Bernáth, 2002).

In particular, transmission of antibodies is a coordinated process between the mother and the newborn and so it is closely connected to reproduction (Baintner, 2007). In vertebrates, a wide range of different reproductive strategies evolved: it can occur pre-partum, via the placenta or yolk sac, or post-partum via ingestion of colostrum and milk.

In avian species, three classes of antibodies are found: IgY, IgA, and IgM. The IgY is the functional equivalent of mammals IgG (the avian IgG counterpart) and is transferred to the yolk to passively protect the developing chick (Kovacs-Nolan & Mine, 2012).

In mammals, IgG is the predominant immunoglobulin isotype in the blood and extravascular space playing an essential role in mediating immunity and it is the main immunoglobulin isotype transferred from the mother to her offspring (Waldmann& Strober, 1969). In fact, maternal passive immunity to several infectious agents is dependent on active IgG transport from mother to newborn or neonate (Baintner, 2007; Cervenak & Kacskovics, 2009; Kacskovics, 2004). In primates and rabbits, maternal IgG is transported through the placenta during fetal life (see Table below). In rodents, as mice and rats, maternal IgG is transmitted both across the yolk sac to the fetus and also postnatal from milk via the neonatal small intestine by a prolonged period, 16 and 21 days respectively (Kacskovics 2004; Baintner 2007; Cervenak and Kacskovics 2009). In dogs and cats the transfer of IgG occurs by a combination of prenatal and postnatal mechanisms, with 5 to 10% of total transfer occurring before birth (Chuma, Hirota, Hasegawa, & Tomoda, 1988; Sidell, RamaRao, Tompkins, & Hansen, 1979; Trowald-Wigh, Ohannisson, & Håkansson, 1993).

In polygastric and monogastric ungulates from the order *Artiodactyla* (ruminants, horses and pigs), fetuses acquire little or no maternal antibodies across the placenta and are born virtually agammaglobulinemic. During colostrum intake, the intestines of these neonates are able to transfer, by non-specific mechanism, immunoglobulins and other macromolecules into the bloodstream. This process takes place for a limited time after birth, generally between 24-36 hours. Later, the intestine suffers a drastic modification named *gut closure*, whereupon immunoglobulins are no longer absorbed from the intestines and they only act locally (Barrington & Parish, 2001).

The cessation of absorption of intact macromolecules, this gut closure, occurs at different ages in different species. In calves and pigs, closure normally occurs by 24-36 hours after birth. During this process, besides cell maturation and tissue replacement in the intestinal mucosa, a gradual transition from the inhibition of proteolysis to the rapid degradation of proteins takes place. Although acquisition of undigested maternal antibodies is essential, the young animal also requires amino acids of proteolytic origin to synthesize its own proteins. This may explain why farm animals limit the absorption of proteins for a short period of time (1–2 days). This limited time is compensated by the efficiency of the absorption, which includes the development of transport vacuoles and the considerable length of the gut. A similar mechanism may function in horses and in carnivores. However, in cats and dogs (Carnivora), shortness of the gut is compensated for by a prenatal, transplacental transmission process (Baintner, 2007).

In particular, immunoglobulin absorption in neonates of large domestic species is aided by the presence of protease inhibitors in the colostrum and its efficiency declines rapidly after birth, with maximal absorption occurring in the first 4 hours (Besser& Gay, 1994; Kehrli & Harp, 2001; Quigley & Drewry, 1998; Salmon, 2000; Stelwagen, Carpenter, Haigh, Hodgkinson, & Wheeler, 2009). The presence of an acid-resistant colostral trypsin inhibitor has been documented in two orders (Artiodactyla and Carnivora) (Baintner, 2007). The trypsin inhibitor contributes to the protection of colostral proteins from proteolysis, but is unable to prevent the full range of pancreatic proteases. The absence of the inhibitor in mare's colostrum shows that its function is not essential. It appears that the high amount of ingested IgG is more important than the protective factor (Baintner & Csapó, 1996).

In 1958, Brambell described a saturable receptor system now called neonatal Fc receptor –FcRn (Junghans, 1997). The FcRs are cell surface molecules that bind the Fc region of immunoglobulins. Each member of the family recognizes immunoglobulin of one isotype or a few closely related isotypes. FcRs can be classified into two functional classes. One class of receptors present on the surfaces of effector cells triggers various biological responses upon binding antibody–antigen complexes. These are the Fcγ receptors for IgG (FcγRI, FcγRII, FcγRIII and the bovine Fcγ2R), the Fcε receptors for IgE (FcεRI, FcεRII), and the Fcα receptor for IgA (FcαRI). The other classes of receptors – the poly IgA receptor (pIgR) and the neonatal IgG transporter (FcRn) – are responsible for the transport of immunoglobulins across epithelial surfaces (Kacskovics, 2004; Ravetch, 1997).

As mentioned, in most livestock species, antibody dependent maternal immunity is exclusively mediated by colostral immunoglobulins and best characterized in ruminants. The presence of bovine FcRn transcripts in multiple tissues, including the mammary gland, suggests their involvement in IgG transcytosis (Kacskovics, Wu, Simister, Frenyo, & Hammarstrom, 2000). In fact, the active transport mediated by FcRn occurs within the cells by transcytosis within clathrin-coated vesicles. The transport is bidirectional and pH-dependent, showing high-affinity binding at acidic pH (pH: 6.5) and weak or no binding at neutral pH (pH: 7.0) (Raghavan, Bonagura, Morrison, & Bjorkman, 1995; Vaughn & Bjorkman, 1998). This pH specificity ensures specific binding in endosomes and the surface of specific cell types (duodenal enterocytes, placental tissue) and the proper release in bloodstream circulation (pH: 7.4). A recent study described the mechanism of FcRn recycling from the endosome to the cell surface in real time and it was seen that the FcRn carries IgG from the recycling endosome to the cell surface and the exocytosis can occur by two pathways: i) classical models of exocytosis of membrane receptors whether the vesicle containing the FcRn fuses completely with the plasma membrane and delivers the FcRn to the cell surface. ii) The kiss-and-run exocytosis where the secretory vesicle remains structurally intact, fusing only partially with the plasma membrane in repetitive cycles, although FcRn can still migrate out of the vesicle to mix with other cell-surface components (Lencer& Blumberg, 2005; R. J. Ober, Martinez, Lai, Zhou, & Ward, 2004; R. Ober, Martinez, Vaccaro, Zhou, & Ward, 2004).

In summary, the complex structure of the ungulate placenta and the lack of FcRn expression on it, determines that the maternal immune transport in ruminants, horses and pigs, is exclusively mediated by colostral intake in a very short period of time after birth. In these species, the transference of antibody from the mother to the offspring is also a dual process of immunoglobulins´ active transport: i) enrichment of maternal lactogenic secretion with isotype specific immunoglobulins by a receptor mediated process, ii) The absorption of this immunoglobulins by the neonate by a non-selective process, iii) IgG re-cycling back to the intestine by a receptor mediated process (Baintner, 2007; Cervenak & Kacskovics, 2009; Kacskovics, 2004).

Regarding the transference of IgY from the hen to the chicks, the yolk sac membranes isolated from chicken, express a functionally equivalent receptor named FcRY with IgY-binding properties similar to those of FcRn for mammalian IgG. The FcRY is structurally homologous to the mammalian MHC family member PLA2R, showing a bidirectional saturable and specific transcytosis of IgY (West, Herr, & Bjorkman, 2004). Co-localization studies showed FcRY-mediated internalization via clathrin-coated pits and transport involving early and recycling endosomes. The binding to IgY is pH-dependent, with high-affinity binding at acidic pH and no observable binding at neutral or basic pH. The FcRY showed a preferred apical-to-basolateral directionality promoting the transport from the apical surface of yolk sac membrane cells (pH:6) to the basolateral surface leading to the circulation of the developing chick (pH:7.4) (Tesar, Cheung, & Bjorkman, 2008).

Species (Taxon)	**Maternal Secretion**	**Absorption by the young**	
		Prenatally	**Postnatally**
Hen/chick *(Aves)*	Across the vitelline membrane surrounding the yolk	Yolk sac endoderm, FcRY	Yolk sac endoderm, FcRY
Opossum *(Theria)*	Secretion into the pouch	No transmission	Small intestine, FrR
Rabbit *(Lagomorpha)*	Uterine epithelium	Everted yolk sac, FcR	No transmission
Rat/mice *(Rodentia)*	Mammary gland (milk), FcRn	Everted yolk sac, FcRn	Proximal small intestine, FcRn
Human *(Primates)*		Placenta and fetal gut, FcRn	No significant transmission
Cattle, sheep and pig *(Artiodactyla)*	Mammary gland (colostrum), FcRn	No transmission	Small intestine, without FcRn
Horse *(Perissodactyla)*	Mammary gland (colostrum)	No transmission	Small intestine
Dog *(Carnivora)*	Mammary gland	Placenta	Small intestine

(Baintner, 2007).

The "Other Side" of the Immunological Connection between Dams and Offspring: Cytokines and Cells

Beside its protective capacity, it has been documented that colostrum has potent immunomodulatory properties and can prevent newborns from mounting active immune responses to specific antigens. Colostrum also has a profound effect on postnatal development of the endogenous immune system and specifically on the B cell lineage (Butler, Zhao, Sinkora, Wertz, & Kacskovics, 2009). Furthermore, colostrum intake can inhibit mucosal and systemic antibody secreting cell production in the newborns, as demonstrated in calves and piglets (Hodgins et al., 1999; Parreño et al., 2004).

Even when immunoglobulins are the main molecules associated with protection, recent studies have revealed that various bioactive components present in colostrum, such as growth and anti-microbial factors are responsible for the immunomodulation of the active neonatal immune response. Growth factors promote the growth and development of the newborn, while anti-microbial factors provide unspecific passive immunity and protect against infections during the first weeks of life (Nguyen et al., 2007; Salmon et al., 2009; Salmon, 2000).

Other maternal immune factors transferred to the neonates include soluble molecules (like growth factors and cytokines) and lymphoid and non-lymphoid cells. Studies in humans showed the transfer of cytokines via the placenta and the components of colostrum/milk. This suggests possible roles for maternal cytokines such as TGF-β, IL-1, IL-6, TNF-α, etc., in immunologic protection of neonates and in modulating neonatal immune development during colonization by commensal bacteria, but did not assess multiple types of cytokines as Th1, Th2, Th3 and T regulatory type 1, or their profiles over time in infants (Bocci et al., 1993).

Various hormones and growth factors, such as insulin, insulin-like growth factors (IGF), epidermal growth factors –EGF- and TGF, have been found in the mammary gland secretions of different species. The most abundant and well-characterized growth factors in bovine colostrum are in fact IGF, insulin, TGF and EGF-(Blum & Baumrucker, 2008; Ginjala & Pakkanen, 1998). In particular, anti-microbial factors in bovine colostrum (besides immunoglobulins) include lactoferrin, lysozyme, lactoperoxidase and a large number of cytokines like IL-2, TNF, IL-1, IL-6 and leukocytes (van Hooijdonk, Kussendrager, & Steijns, 2000).

Several studies have also investigated the potential of milk proteins to affect lymphocyte function after *in vivo* exposure and have suggested a degree of immunoenhancement of lymphocyte function due to various components, including some nonspecific products (like casein), pro-inflammatory cytokines (IL-1b, IL-6, TNF-α and IFN-γ) or growth factors (EGF and TGF-α) present in bovine colostrum (Cross & Gill, 1999, 2000). The concentrations of these bioactive compounds are usually high in colostrum, decline rapidly in mature milk and are often below the detection level in infant formula or colostrum and milk replacers. For example, TGF-β concentration in porcine colostrum collected at the time of parturition ranged between 126 and 260 ng/ml; it declined to 72 ng/ml 12 hours after parturition, and became undetectable in milk collected 5 days after parturition (Xu et al., 1999). Natural suckling or oral feeding with porcine or bovine colostrum significantly reduced the staining intensity of TGF-β receptors in the jejunal and ileal villous epithelium of the small intestine in newborn pigs suggesting that colostrum-borne TGF-β modulates intestinal function in suckling animals (R. Xu, Wang, & Zhang, 2000).

Other components, such as lactoferrin, whey proteins or lactoperoxidase, may have the opposite effect by inhibiting the induction of IL-2 or by the presence of the colostrum inhibitory factors, which inhibits the induction of IL-2 in human T lymphocytes (Cross & Gill, 2000; Mandalapu, Pabst, & Paetkau, 1995; Sfeir, Dubarry, Boyaka, Rautureau, & Tomé, 2004).

These reports provide strong evidence that bovine colostrum, with its multiple components, is able to modulate lymphocyte function in several different ways. The role of cytokines in the regulation and modulation of the immune response has been studied extensively in the past. Cytokines are produced by different Th CD4+ cells (Th1, Th2, Th3 and Tr1 types). IFN-γ and IL-12 are produced by Th1 cells and they promote inflammatory and cytotoxic T lymphocyte responses. IL-4 and IL-5 are produced by Th2 cells and they promote B cell responses. TGF-β is produced mainly by Th3 cells that have immunoregulatory functions. IL-10 is produced by Th2 and Tr1 cells and plays an important role in antibody production and in anti-inflammatory responses (Foussat et al., 2003).

Bovine colostrum shows an immunomodulatory effect mainly targeting the gut-associated lymphoid tissues, which respond by producing both Th1 and Th2 cytokines. This bipolarity is important in the context of exposure to a wide range of antigens associated with pathogens, with commensal bacteria and with food and includes the ability to generate tolerance to food and commensal bacterial antigens as well as to activate the immune response to pathogens causing danger in the mucosa (Boudry et al., 2007). An important practical consequence of these immunosuppressive effects is that colostrum fed animals have impaired antibody responses to natural infection as well as vaccination compared to colostrum-deprived animals (Hodgins et al., 1999; Nguyen et al., 2007; Parreño et al., 1999, 2004).

The presence of these cytokines in mammary secretions likely influences development of the neonatal immune system. Of the maternal cytokines, TGF-β has been experimentally studied extensively in humans, mice and rats. In mammals, three isoforms of TGF-β (β1, β2 and β3) have been identified of which TGF-β1 is the most abundant form in tissues whereas TGF-β2 is more abundant in body fluids (Miyazono, Ichijo, & Heldin, 1993). Porcine milk contains abundant TGF-β, which was suggested to play a role in regulating the intestinal immune system in neonatal pigs. In this vein of research, Nguyen and colleagues extended the research and evaluated the concentrations and number of cells secreting various pro-inflammatory (IL-6 and TNF-α), Th1 (IFN-γ and IL-12), Th2 (IL-4 and IL-10) and Th3 (TGF-β) cytokines in sow serum, colostrum and milk. They studied the transfer and persistence of maternal cytokines in neonates and also examined the functions of porcine TGF-β and IL-4 on naïve and antigen activated-B cells in vitro. This study showed a high concentration of IL-4, followed by TGF-β1, similar concentrations of IL-6 and IFN-γ, moderate concentration of IL-12 and low concentrations of IL-10 and TNF-α in colostrum/milk of conventional sows. The cytokine concentration in lactogenic secretions were generally correlated with their respective concentrations in sow serum except for TGF-β1, which was higher high in colostrum/milk and the TNF-α, which was detected in colostrum/milk and was absent in sow serum. These results suggested that most of cytokines found in colostrum and milk might be transported from the circulation to the mammary secretions while the high concentration of TGF-β1 and TNF-α suggested that these two cytokines were produced locally in the mammary gland. The study done by Nguyen et al. in 2007 in newborn pigs also demonstrated that after colostrum intake, and prior to gut closure, there was transference of maternal cytokines into the bloodstream circulation of the piglets (except for TNF-α; IL-12 and TGF-β1). TNF-α was not transferred, while the detection of IL-12 and TGF-β1 in pre-suckling and colostrum-deprived gnotobiotic piglet serum suggested the constitutive production of these two cytokines, however the other cytokines were undetectable prior to suckling confirming the absence of transplacental transfer. The authors documented the transference and persistence of maternal cytokines from colostrum/milk to neonates and speculated that cytokine concentration in piglet sera could be attributed not only to the absorption of cytokines present in colostrum but also to the cytokine produced by the colostral cells that can be transferred to the piglet across the intestinal epithelium (Nguyen et al., 2007; Tuboly & Bernáth, 2002).

Similar findings were reported in bovine colostrum where cytokine mRNAs of IL-1β, IL-6, TNF-β and INF-γ were detected by RT-PCR in the colostrum cells. The concentrations of these cytokines measured by ELISA were significantly higher in colostrum than in the mature milk. These cytokines were detected in sera of newborn calves, after colostrum intake, reaching peak levels by 24 hours and then gradually decreasing to become undetectable by 4 weeks after birth (Hagiwara, Kataoka, Yamanaka, Kirisawa, & Iwai, 2000; Yamanaka, Hagiwara, Kirisawa, & Iwai, 2003).

However, the immune system always acts coordinately. The studies conducted in pigs together with work conducted in cattle, mice and humans, indicate that IL-4 and TGF-β play a critical role in isotype switching to IgA and in the production of secretory IgA antibodies, which function in immune exclusion of bacterial and viral pathogens and by their coating of commensals, may limit the penetration of commensals beyond the intestinal epithelium (Lencer & Blumberg, 2005; Nguyen et al., 2007). Thus, the high concentrations of TGF-β1 and IL-4 in the colostrum/milk may play an important immunoregulatory role in the intestinal mucosa of the neonates, like establishment and maintenance of the initial commensal microflora in the intestine and promotion of secretory IgA responses needed to maintain gut homeostasis and tolerance to dietary antigens (Bailey et al., 2007; Iijima, Takahashi, & Kiyono, 2001; Lencer & Blumberg, 2005).

Experimental evidence indicates that ingestion of colostrum is also important in postnatal adaptation of the newborn gastrointestinal tract, particularly stimulating intestinal cell growth (Guilloteau, Zabielski, & Blum, 2009). Colostrum modulates postnatal gastrointestinal adaptation by altering intestinal TGF-β receptor intensity in newborn pigs. It has been demonstrated that villous height and crypt depth were significantly greater in piglets fed with porcine or bovine colostrum than in piglets fed with porcine milk, infant formula or water. The molecular mechanisms involved in these processes are believed to be mediated by various bioactive compounds in the colostrum (R. Xu et al., 2000).

Passive Immunity Strategies against Enteric Diseases in Calves

Taking advantage of this natural process, vaccination of the dams has become a well-established practice among veterinary practitioners in order to increase the levels of passive maternal antibodies transferred from the mother to her offspring to prevent neonatal diseases. This strategy of passive systemic immunity has been applied with optimal results, especially for systemic infections. In cattle, dams are vaccinated at least 3 weeks pre-partum in order

to raise antigen-specific antibodies that would later be transferred passively in colostrum to the newborn. The application of systematic vaccination of the dam in the late stage of pregnancy increases the levels of specific immunoglobulins in serum and colostrums (Saif & Fernandez, 1996).

The systematic application of vaccine to promote passive immunity against enteric disease, although reducing diarrhea morbidity, showed variable efficacy (Bellinzoni et al., 1989). As an example, while a significant reduction in duration and diarrhea severity occurred in calves fed once shortly after birth with pooled immune colostrum from cows immunized against bovine rotavirus, only limited protection against viral challenge was observed (Parreño et al., 2004). The variable success of maternal rotavirus vaccines in the market is influenced by vaccine dose, strain, inactivating agent, adjuvant, route of administration, and environmental rotavirus exposure levels (Saif & Fernandez, 1996).

The use of intramammary route together with genetically engineered rotavirus-like particle (VLP) vaccines in cows to boost antibodies in mammary secretions showed promising results demonstrating a significant increase of antibody titer in colostrum and milk and high protection rates in calves (Fernandez et al., 1996). Such subunit vaccines possess potential advantages over existing vaccines. An effort to reduce the cost of scaling up the VLP technology for veterinary vaccine production is under progress (Liu et al., 2013). The development of delivery system to the mammary gland will help to adopt this excellent route into the routine practice in dairy cows.

A key concept regarding vaccines to prevent enteric mucosal infections is that the induced immunity is not sterilizing, as can happen for systemic infections like the vaccination against Food and Mouth Disease. So far, the best scenario for a vaccine to an enteric pathogen would be that suckling animals born to vaccinated mothers become sub-clinically infected while receiving adequate passive antibodies to prevent the disease and develop active immunity (natural attenuation induced by passive maternal antibodies) (Fernandez et al., 1996; Nguyen et al., 2006; Parreño et al., 2004; Saif & Fernandez, 1996). This balance between passive immunity and disease can easily be disrupted in intensive animal production systems by exposing animals to high pathogen doses in confined, contaminated environments. In addition, earlier weaning practices, with feeding of supplements or milk replacers curtail or dilute milk antibodies. Consequently, without maternal vaccines, antibody titers to enteric pathogens usually decrease to un-protective levels in milk. Even in vaccinated dams the antibody titers in milk decrease sharply after calving, as depicted in Figure 1, where vaccinated cows were monitored to study the evolution of IgG1 antibody titers to rotavirus (RVA) in serum, colostrums and milk after vaccination. The anti-RVA IgG1 transferred to their calves was evident, as they showed similar Ab titers in serum to that detected in the colostrum of their dams. IgG1 Ab titer to RVA was also detected in calves' feces. The IgG1 Ab titer to RVA decreases sharply from colostrum to mature milk as well as in calves' feces until unprotected levels, at three weeks of age, the moment of peak RVA diarrhea incidence in the herd (Parreño and Marcoppido, unpublished data).

On the other hand, failure of passive transfer (FPT) is a common problem in newborn calves and even more frequent in newborn foals (Becvarova & Buechner-Maxwell, 2012; Besser & Gay, 1994; Nath, Anderson, Savage, & McKinnon, 2010). The FPT is a well-established cause of increase of neonatal morbidity and mortality associated with intestinal, respiratory and systemic diseases and the single most important predisposing factor for development of neonatal septicemia in foals and calves. Mortality of dairy calves born alive from birth to weaning is greater than 10% in the U.S. Approximately 50% of mortality that occurred in pre-weaned calves is directly related to inadequate acquisition of passive immunity (Quigley & Drewry, 1998).

Evaluation of passive transfer of colostrum antibodies in the foal's and calf´s serum should be performed in order to confirm proper absorption. This measure is normally done between 12 to 24 hours after birth. If the level is not adequate, early detection of FPT allows administration of colostrum (or other immunoglobulin supplementation) within an optimal window of time. The best ways to measure immunoglobulin´s concentration in newborn are the radial immune diffusion (RID) and ELISA tests (Erhard, Luft, Remler, & Stangassinger, 2001). It has been reported that immunoglobulin concentrations between 1 g/L and 8 g/L in serum are protective levels against death from septicemia, while higher levels between 7.5 g/L and 16 g/L are needed for protection against neonatal diarrhea in calves. An immunoglobulin concentration of 10 g/L is accepted as an optimal level of passive transference (Waldner & Rosengren, 2009).

This FPT of maternal immunoglobulins involves maternal, calf, environmental and management factors. The age, number of parturitions and breed of the mother are important factors associated to FPT. The presence of mastitis and agalactia led to a failure of the dam to produce good quality colostrum, resulting in inadequate levels of maternal antibodies. Dams can also suffer leakage of colostrum prior to parturition. Regarding newborns, a delay to suckle colostrum within the first 4-6 hours of life (the highest immunoglobulins absorption), the ingestion of low quantities of colostrum or inefficient absorption in the gut, are reason for FPT. Environmental factors such as cold weather or heat stress affect both mother and newborn, preventing them from reaching optimal levels of passive transference. Finally, management factors such as vaccination, hygiene, control of immunoglobulin levels, and administration of colostrum replacers as well as immune milks are important tools to reduce FPT (Besser & Gay, 1994; Waldner & Rosengren, 2009).

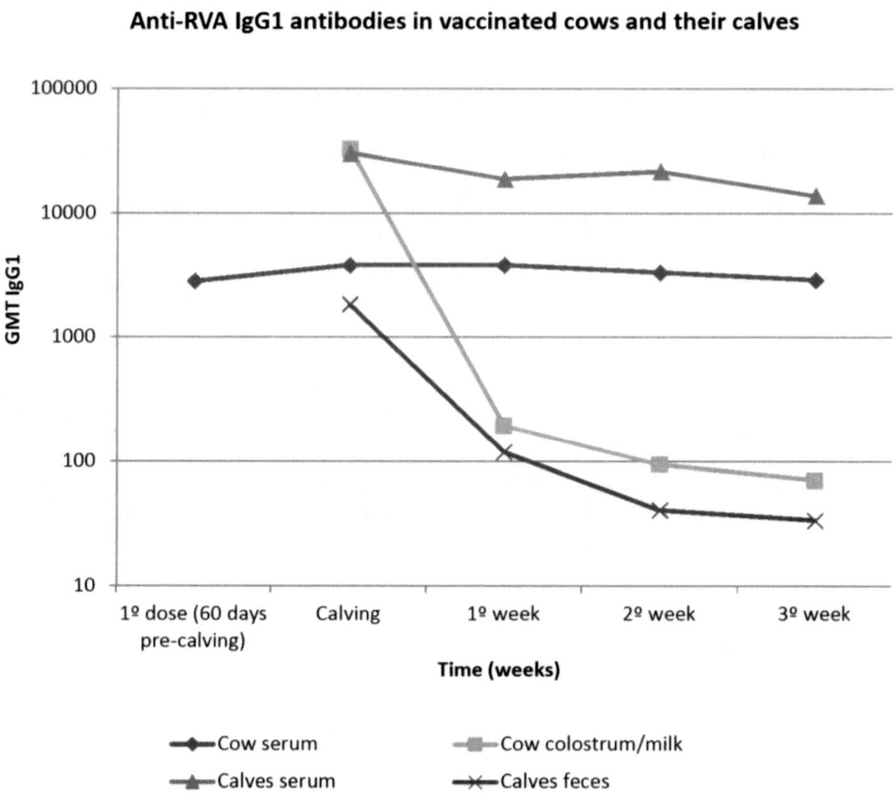

Figure 1. Anti-RVA IgG1 Ab titer in serum, colostrum and milk of cows vaccinated with a RVA vaccine, 60 and 30 days before calving. Anti RVA IgG1 transferred to their calves after colostrum intake in serum and feces. Geometric mean titer (GMT) of 10 animals.

This problem led to the development of other alternative and/or complementary passive local immunity strategies based on the production of immune milks supplemented with homologous and heterologous antibodies to different enteropathogens. Our group of research has been focused in the development of prevention strategies against rotavirus diarrhea in calves (Parreno, Marcoppido et al. 2010; Vega, Bok et al. 2011). The efficacy of this treatment is studied in a calf model of rotavirus infection and disease (Figure 2). The timing for oral artificial administration of colostrum or colostrum replacers is critical (within 6 hours after birth). After that, intravenous administration of plasma is often considered to provide passive transfer of immunoglobulins to the newborns (Nath et al., 2010; Quigley & Drewry, 1998).

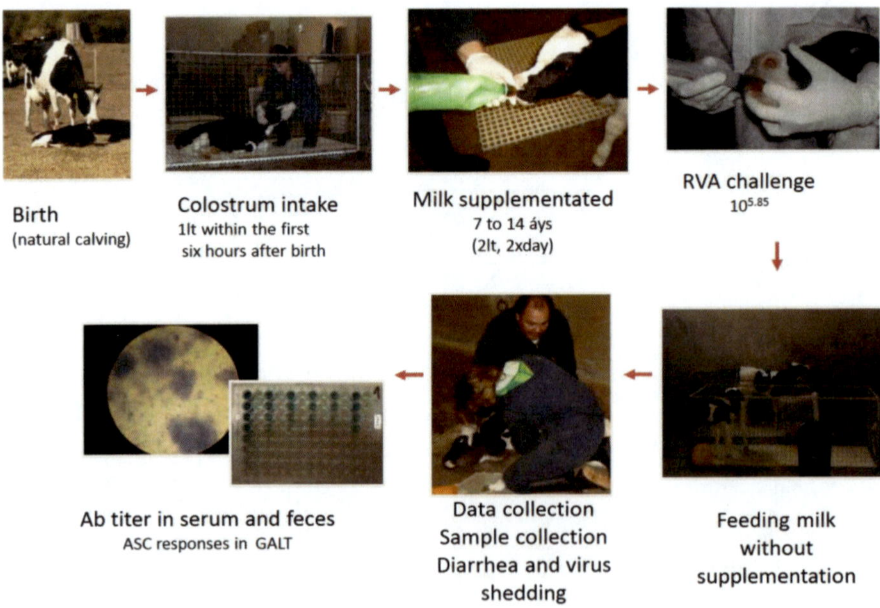

Figure 2. Neonatal calf model of Rotavirus infection and disease.

Passive Immunity Strategies Based in Homologous Antibodies

Different sources of antibody (i.e., oral administration of hyperimmune plasma; fluid or powdered bovine immune colostrum, fluid or powdered chicken egg yolk enriched in IgY polyclonal antibodies) have been explored. Most of these strategies represent effective immunotherapies to prevent gastrointestinal infections in animals and some of them are commercially available. Other approaches are still under evaluation.

Numerous commercial immunoglobulin preparations with activity against specific enteric pathogens have been marketed over the last several decades. Products intended for prevention of *Escherichia coli* enteritis in calves include dried bovine colostrum and whey, hyperimmune sera raised in horses, and mouse monoclonal antibodies to the K99 (F5) antigen of E. coli. These products are administered orally in the first 12 hours of life to prevent adhesion of enteropathogenic *E. coli*. Bovine immunoglobulin products containing antibodies to antigens of *E. coli* pathogenic for neonatal pigs have also been marketed for oral use in piglets. Orally administered bovine colostral whey containing rotavirus antibodies also passively protected piglets (in the absence of circulating antibodies) in a dose dependent manner, but did not interfere with induction of active serum antibody responses (Cordle et al., 1991).

The immunomodulatory effect caused by the administration of milk supplemented with immune colostrum on the systemic and mucosal humoral immune responses was investigated in newborn calves experimentally infected with bovine rotavirus (Parreño, et al., 2010). This study evaluated the protection and immune modulation after a first exposure to bovine rotavirus at 2 days of age followed by a second challenge after the cessation of feeding supplemented milk in conventional calves. The administration of the supplemented milk twice a day, for 14 days, resembles management practices in dairy farms, where farmers collect the colostrum of dairy cows and use it to supplement the diet of calves under artificial rearing. The supplementation of milk diets with immune colostrum induced protection against rotavirus diarrhea after inoculation in a dose-dependent manner. This protection was associated with the presence of passive IgG1 in the feces of these calves. A final IgG1 antibody titer to bovine rotavirus of 1/4096 (0.8% of fed volume) induced 80% protection against rotavirus diarrhea and 40% protection against virus shedding, after inoculation. The animals also showed full protection against diarrhea after a second exposure to the virus (7 days after the end of the passive treatment). The results indicated that passive antibody treatment for 14 days was effective in protecting most of the animals during the entire period of susceptibility to rotavirus infection (Figure 3). The treatment significantly suppressed active systemic antibody responses in terms of antibody titers in serum modifying the isotype profile of the active antibody responses toward higher IgA than IgM, reduced the antibody secreting cell -ASC- responses in blood, spleen and mesenteric lymph nodes (Parreño V et al., 2010).

Similar results were reported in gnotobiotic pigs vaccinated with human rotavirus, in the presence of passive circulating antibodies (Nguyen et al., 2006) and infected in the presences of circulating and local passive maternal antibodies (Hodgins et al., 1999).

In contrast to the suppressive effect at the systemic level, the supplementation of milk with bovine rotavirus-immune colostrum enhanced and diversified the profile of the ASC responses in the intestinal mucosa, toward higher numbers of IgA ASC in the proximal intestinal mucosa and increasing numbers of IgG2 ASC. The ASC response to a second exposure to the virus in the absence of passive antibodies, was characterized by high and similar numbers of IgA and IgG1 and IgG2, indicating that for calves, IgG is also an important effector at the mucosal sites. The immune suppression effect observed in systemic tissues and the positive immunomodulation in the intestinal mucosa agreed with the studies conducted by Nguyen and colleagues regarding the suppressive effect of a high concentration of maternal cytokines transferred to the newborn circulation after colostrum intake and the positive effect of the same biomolecules in lower concentration acting locally in the gut (Nguyen et al., 2007).

Oral Administration of Chicken Egg Yolk Antibodies - IgY

Immunization of chickens shows promise as an efficient method to produce polyclonal antibodies for passive protection. Specific antibodies of the IgYisotype are induced by vaccination and are concentrated in egg yolk. Laying hens can produce about 20 g of IgY per year. Thus, hens' eggs are an excellent source of large quantities of antibodies that can be used for passive immunization applications, not only for chickens but also for other veterinary species and also human infants. This technology has been tested against a number of pathogens for different syndromes, including bursal disease virus, avian coccidiosis, bovine rotavirus and coronavirus, porcine epidemic diarrhea virus, canine parvovirus-2, enterotoxigenic *E. coli*, *Salmonella* sp. in cattle and pigs, prevention of respiratory diseases and mastitis in cattle, and as passive treatment in aquaculture among other uses (Kovacs-Nolan & Mine, 2012; Mine & Kovacs-Nolan, 2002; Sarker, Pant, Juneja, & Hammarström, 2007; Schade et al., 2005; Tini, Jewell, Camenisch, Chilov, & Gassmann, 2002; Y Xu et al., 2011). Several of these IgY products are commercially made.

Besides its proved effectiveness for passive protection, a recent study has shown the immunomodulatory effect induced by the oral administration of milk supplemented with crude egg yolk in neonatal calves challenged with bovine rotavirus (Vega et al., 2011). The study showed that supplementing the diets of newborn calves with rotavirus-specific IgY for the first 14 days of life induces up to 80% protection against diarrhea after challenge. Later on, a spray dried IgY preparation was used for therapeutic treatment of rotavirus-infected calves. This treatment was maintained for 7 consecutive days once diarrhea appeared and significantly reduced clinical symptoms (Vega et al., in press).

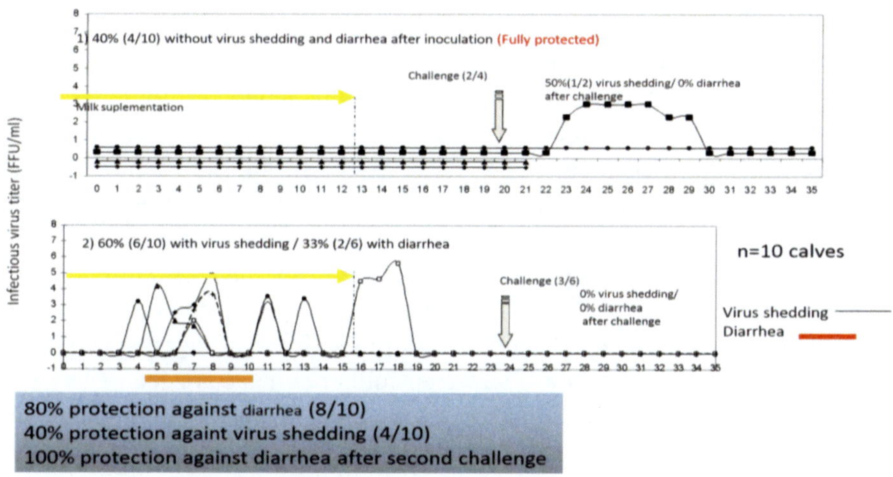

Figure 3. Calves fed control colostrum (RVA IgG1= 16,384) + milk supplemented with colostrum with a final Ab titer to RVA 4096. Modified from Parreño et al., 2010.

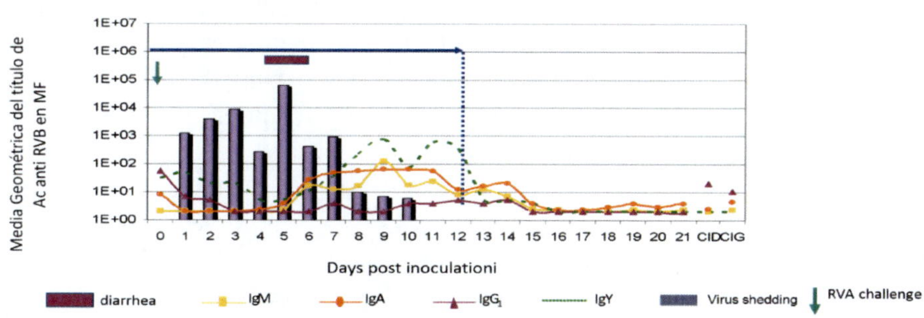

Calves fed control colostrum (RVA IgG1 16,384 + milk supplemented with RVA IgY 4096 14 days (n = 5). Modified from Veja et al., 2011.

Figure 4. Protection against RVA diarrhea in calves fed milk supplemented with egg yolk enriched in IgY to RVA.

More importantly, calves fed milk supplemented with chicken egg yolk showed a significant diversification and enhancement of the mucosal ASC responses against rotavirus infection. Interestingly, this effect was independent of the specificity of the treatment and was significantly more pronounced than the one induced with bovine immune colostrum (Parreño, et al., 2010; Vega, et al., 2011). These results are in agreement with the presence of bioactive immunomodulatory molecules (hormones, cytokines, lysophosphatidylcholine, etc.) in egg yolks, that have been shown to promote B cell clonal expansion and IgA switching related to anti-inflammatory responses to dietary antigens (Nelson, Katayamab, Mine, Duarte, & Matar, 2007; YP Xu et al., 2006).

Further research where protection against rotavirus diarrhea conferred by the prophylactic administration of specific IgY antibodies to gnotobiotic piglets experimentally inoculated with a human strain of rotavirus was conducted. Supplementation for 9 days conferred full protection against diarrhea and significantly reduced virus shedding. This protection was dose-dependent. However, the oral administration of semi-purified passive IgY from chickens did not affect the isotype profile of the pig ASC responses to rotavirus infection, but it was associated with significantly fewer numbers of specific IgA ASC in the duodenum. In this study, the pigs' immune responses to the passive IgY treatment were further characterized. The oral administration of IgY induced IgGAb responses to chicken IgY in serum and local IgA and IgGAb responses to IgY in the intestinal contents of neonatal piglets in a dose dependent manner (Vega et al., 2012).

It seems like this strategy based on IgY antibodies can be scaled-up to inexpensively produce large amounts of polyclonal immunoglobulins from egg yolks to be applied as a preventive and therapeutic passive treatment to control diarrhea. A better understanding of the immunomodulatory effects of egg yolk on the immune system of heterologous species will expand the use of the IgY technology not only as a passive immune strategy for disease preventive but also as a specific disease therapy (treatment).

Final Considerations

Maternal vaccination to enhance passive immunity is already widely used in veterinary medicine. Some of these vaccines, especially conventional vaccines against enteric viruses, have limited efficacy and FPT is a common event in livestock newborn animals. However, new approaches to enhance immunogenicity have been successful and they are being scaled up, so these new technologies will become economically viable in the near future.

Commercial products have already been developed as supplements for newborns that have received inadequate amounts or quality of colostrum. The new understanding of the mechanisms behind protection and immunomodulation will span its rationale use. The ability to provide continuity of immune protection from birth, by combining homologous and heterologous antibody sources for passive immunity with active immunization would have a major impact on neonatal morbidity and mortality.

On the other hand, passive immunity has been documented to often interfere with newborn active immune responses to natural infections and vaccination. In the recent years, the transference of immune cells and other biomolecules with immunomodulatory properties from the mother to the offspring had been described as clarifying the mechanisms behind this interference. New adjuvants, antigen delivery systems and rationale vaccine designs to overwhelm or take advantage of the properties of these passive maternal biomolecules and cells transferred to the newborns are under development. Various factors affect and modulate the infant gut mucosal immune system: components of the intestinal barrier, the infant gut microbiome, nutrition and the maternal-infant hybrid immune system. Elucidation of the phenotypic distribution of immune cells, their functional significance and the mucosa-specific pathways used by these cells is essential to the future of research in the field of infant immunology (Battersby & Gibbons, 2013).

References

Bailey, M., Haverson, K., Inman, C., Harris, C., Jones, P., Corfield, G., … & Stokes, C. (2007). The development of the mucosal immune system pre- and post-weaning: balancing regulatory and effector function. *Proceedings of the Nutrition Society*, *64*(04), 451–457. doi:10.1079/PNS2005452

Baintner, K. (2007). Transmission of antibodies from mother to young: Evolutionary strategies in a proteolytic environment. *Veterinary Immunology and Immunopathology*, *117*(3-4), 153–61. doi:10.1016/j.vetimm.2007.03.001

Baintner, K. & Csapó, J. (1996). Lack of acid-resistant trypsin inhibitor in mare's colostrum: short communication. *Acta Veterinaria Hungarica, 44*(1), 95–7.

Bandrick, M., Ariza-Nieto, C., Baidoo, S. & Molitora, T. (2014). Colostral antibody-mediated and cell-mediated immunity contributes to innate and antigen-specific immunity in piglets. *Developmental & Comparative Immunology*, *43*(1), 114–120.

Barrington, G. & Parish, S. (2001). Bovine neonatal immunology. *Vet Clin North Am Food Anim Pract.*, *17*(3), 463–76.

Battersby, A. J. & Gibbons, D. L. (2013). The gut mucosal immune system in the neonatal period. *Pediatr Allergy Immunol*, *24*, 414–421.

Becvarova, I. & Buechner-Maxwell, V. (2012). Feeding the foal for immediate and long-term health. *Equine Veterinary Journal*, *41*(supplement), 149–56.

Bellinzoni, R., Blackhall, J., Baro, N., Auza, N., Mattion, N., Casaro, A., … &Scodeller, E. (1989). Efficacy of an inactivated oil-adjuvanted rotavirus vaccine in the control of calf diarrhea in beef herds in Argentina. *Vaccine*, *7*(3), 263–8.

Besser, T. & Gay, C. (1994). The importance of colostrum to the health of the neonatal calf. *The Veterinary Clinics of North America. Food Animal Practice*, 10(1), 107–17.

Blum, J. & Baumrucker, C. (2008). Insulin-like growth factors (IGFs), IGF binding proteins, and other endocrine factors in milk: role in the newborn. *Advances in Experimental Medicine and Biology*, *606*, 397–422.

Bocci, V., von Bremen, K., Corradeschi, F., Franchi, F., Luzzi, E. & Paulesu, L. (1993). Presence of interferon-gamma and interleukin-6 in colostrum of normal women. *Lymphokine and Cytokine Research*, *12*(1), 21–24.

Boudry, C., Buldgen, A., Portetelle, D., Collard, A., Théwis, A. & Dehoux, J. (2007). Effects of oral supplementation with bovine colostrum on the immune system of weaned piglets. *Research in Veterinary Science*, *83*(1), 91–101.

Butler, J., Zhao, Y., Sinkora, M., Wertz, N. & Kacskovics, I. (2009). Immunoglobulins, antibody repertoire and B cell development. *Developmental & Comparative Immunology*, *33*(3), 321–33.

Cervenak, J. & Kacskovics, I. (2009). The neonatal Fc receptor plays a crucial role in the metabolism of IgG in livestock animals. *Veterinary Immunology and Immunopathology*, *128*(1-3), 171–7. doi:10.1016/j.vetimm.2008.10.300

Chatthaa, K., Vlasovaa, A., Kandasamya, S., Esseilia, M., Siegismund, C., Rajashekara, G. & Saif, L. (2014). Probiotics and colostrum/milk differentially affect neonatal humoral immune responses to oral rotavirus vaccine.*Vaccine*,*31*(15),1916–1923. doi:10.1016/j.vaccine.2013.02.020.Probiotics

Chuma, T., Hirota, Y., Hasegawa, A. & Tomoda, I. (1988). IgG-Fc-receptor positive and negative T cells from feline leukemia virus-infected cats. *Nihon Juigaku Zasshi*, *50*(3), 699–705.

Conrath, K., Wernery, U., Muyldermans, S. & Nguyen, V. (2003). Emergence and evolution of functional heavy-chain antibodies in Camelidae. *Developmental & Comparative Immunology*, *27*(2), 87–102.

Cordle, C., Schaller, J., Winship, T., Candler, E., Hilty, M., Smith, K., … & Krakowka, S. (1991). Passive immune protection from diarrhea caused by rotavirus or *E. coli*: an animal model to demonstrate and quantitate efficacy. *Advances in Experimental Medicine and Biology*, *310*, 317–27.

Cross, M. & Gill, H. (1999). Modulation of immune function by a modified bovine whey protein concentrate. *Immunology and Cell Biology*, *77*, 345–350.

Cross, M. & Gill, H. (2000). Immunomodulatory properties of milk. *British Journal of Nutrition*, *84* (suppl 1), 81–9.

De Meyer, T., Muyldermans, S. & Depicker, A. (2014). Nanobody-based products as research and diagnostic tools. *Trends in Biotechnology*, 32(5), 263–270.

Erhard, M., Luft, C., Remler, H. & Stangassinger, M. (2001). Assessment of colostral transfer and systemic availability of immunoglobulin G in new-born foals using a newly developed enzyme-linked immunosorbent assay (ELISA) system. *Journal of Animal Physiology and Animal Nutrition*, 85(5-6), 164–73.

Fernandez, F., Conner, M., Parwani, A., Todhunter, D., Smith, K., Crawford, S., … & Saif, L. (1996). Isotype-specific antibody responses to rotavirus and virus proteins in cows inoculated with subunit vaccines composed of recombinant SA11 rotavirus core-like particles (CLP) or virus-like particles (VLP). *Vaccine*, *14*(14), 1303–12.

Foussat, A., Cottrez, F., Brun, V., Fournier, N., Breittmayer, J. & Groux, H. (2003). A Comparative Study between T Regulatory Type 1 and CD4 + CD25 + T Cells in the Control of Inflammation. *Journal of Immunology*, *171*(10), 5018–26. doi:10.4049/jimmunol.171.10.5018

Garaicoechea, L., Olichon, A., Marcoppido, G., Wigdorovitz, A., Mozgovoj, M., Saif, L., … & Parreño, V. (2008). Llama-derived single-chain antibody fragments directed to rotavirus VP6 protein possess broad neutralizing activity in vitro and confer protection against diarrhea in mice. *Journal of Virology*, *82*(19), 9753–64.

Ginjala, V. & Pakkanen, R. (1998). Determination of transforming growth factor-beta 1 (TGF-beta 1) and insulin-like growth factor (IGF-1) in bovine colostrum samples. *Journal of Immunoassay*, 19(2-3), 195–207.

Guilloteau, P., Zabielski, R. & Blum, J. (2009). Gastrointestinal tract and digestion in the young ruminant: ontogenesis, adaptations, consequences and manipulations. *Journal of Physiology and Pharmacology : An Official Journal of the Polish Physiological Society*, *60 Suppl 3*, 37–46. Retrieved from http://www.ncbi.nlm.nih.gov/pubmed/19996480

Hagiwara, K., Kataoka, S., Yamanaka, H., Kirisawa, R. & Iwai, H. (2000). Detection of cytokines in bovine colostrum. *Veterinary Immunology and Immunopathology*, *76*(3-4), 183–90.

Hamers-Casterman, C., Tarhouch, T., Muyldermans, S., Robinson, G., Hamers, C., Songa, E., ... & Hamers, R. (1993). Naturally occurring antibodies devoid of light chains. *Nature*, *363*(6428), 446–8.

Hammer, D. & Mossmann, H. (1978). The importance of membrane receptors in the transfer of immunoglobulins from plasma to the colostrum. *Annals of Veterinary Research*, *9*(2), 229–234.

Hodgins, D., Kang, S., DeArriba, L., Parreño, V., Ward, L., Yuan, L., ... & Saif, L. J. (1999). Effects of Maternal Antibodies on Protection and Development of Antibody Responses to Human Rotavirus in Gnotobiotic Pigs Effects of Maternal Antibodies on Protection and Development of Antibody Responses to Human Rotavirus in Gnotobiotic Pigs. *Journal of Virology*, *73*(1), 186–97.

Holt, P. G. & Jones, C. a. (2000). The development of the immune system during pregnancy and early life. *Allergy*, *55*(8), 688–97. Retrieved from http://www.ncbi.nlm.nih.gov/pubmed/10955693

Iijima, H., Takahashi, I. & Kiyono, H. (2001). Mucosal immune network in the gut for the control of infectious diseases. *Reviews in Medical Virology*, *11*(2), 117–33.

Junghans, R. (1997). Finally! The Brambell receptor (FcRB). Mediator of transmission of immunity and protection from catabolism for IgG. *Immunol Res.*, *16*(1), 29–57.

Kacskovics, I. (2004). Fc receptors in livestock species. *Veterinary Immunology and Immunopathology*, *102*(4), 351–62. doi:10.1016/j.vetimm.2004.06.008

Kacskovics, I., Wu, Z., Simister, N. E., Frenyo, L. V. & Hammarstrom, L. (2000). Cloning and Characterization of the Bovine MHC Class I-Like Fc Receptor. *The Journal of Immunology*, *164*(4), 1889–1897. doi:10.4049/ jimmunol.164.4.1889

Kehrli, M. J. & Harp, J. (2001). Immunity in the mammary gland. *The Veterinary Clinics of North America. Food Animal Practice*, *17*(3), 495–516.

Kelly, D. & Coutts, a G. (2000). Early nutrition and the development of immune function in the neonate. *The Proceedings of the Nutrition Society*, *59*(2),177–85 Retrieved from http://www.ncbi.nlm.nih.gov/ pubmed/10946785

Kovacs-Nolan, J. & Mine, Y. (2012). Egg Yolk Antibodies for Passive Immunity. *Annual Review of Food Science and Technology*, 3(163-182).

Lencer, W. & Blumberg, R. (2005). A passionate kiss, then run: exocytosis and recycling of IgG by FcRn. *Trends in Cell Biology*, 15(1), 5–9.

Liu, F., Wu, X., Li, L., Ge, S., Liu, Z. & Wang, Z. (2013). Comp Immunol Microbiol Infect Dis. 2013 Jul;36(4):343-52. doi: 10.1016/j.cimid.2013.02.002. Epub 2013 Apr 3. Virus-like particles: promising platforms with characteristics of DIVA for veterinary vaccine design. *Comparative Immunology, Microbiology and Infectious Diseases*, 36(4), 343–52.

M'Rabet, L., Vos, A., Boehm, G. & Garssen, J. (2008). Breast-feeding and its role in early development of the immune system in infants: consequences for health later in life. *The Journal of Nutrition*, *138*(9), 1782S–1790S. Retrieved from http://www.ncbi.nlm.nih.gov/pubmed/18716187

Mandalapu, P., Pabst, H. & Paetkau, V. (1995). A novel immunosuppressive factor in human colostrum. *Cell Immunology*, 162(2), 178–84.

Mine, Y. & Kovacs-Nolan, J. (2002). Chicken egg yolk antibodies as therapeutics in enteric infectious disease: a review. *Journal of Medical Food*, *5*(3), 159–69.

Miyazono, K., Ichijo, H. & Heldin, C. (1993). Transforming growth factor-beta: latent forms, binding proteins and receptors. *Growth Factors*, *8*(1), 11–22.

Nath, L., Anderson, G., Savage, C. & McKinnon, A. (2010). Use of stored equine colostrum for the treatment of foals perceived to be at risk for failure of transfer of passive immunity. *Journal of the American Veterinary Medical Association*, 236(10), 1085–90.

Nelson, R., Katayamab, S., Mine, Y., Duarte, J. & Matar, C. (2007). Immunomodulating effects of egg yolk low lipid peptic digests in a murine model. *Food and Agricultural Immunology*, 18(1), 1–15.

Nguyen, T., Yuan, L., Azevedo, M., Jeong, K., Gonzalez, A., Iosef, C., … & Saif, L. (2006). Low titer maternal antibodies can both enhance and suppress B cell responses to a combined live attenuated human rotavirus and VLP-ISCOM vaccine. *Vaccine*, *24*(13), 2302–16.

Nguyen, T., Yuan, L., Azevedo, M., Jeong, K., Gonzalez, A. & Saif, L. (2007). Transfer of maternal cytokines to suckling piglets: in vivo and in vitro models with implications for immunomodulation of neonatal immunity. *Veterinary Immunology and Immunopathology*, *117*(3-4), 236–48. doi:10.1016/j.vetimm.2007.02.013

Ober, R. J., Martinez, C., Lai, X., Zhou, J. & Ward, E. S. (2004). Exocytosis of IgG as mediated by the receptor, FcRn: an analysis at the single-molecule level. *Proceedings of the National Academy of Sciences of the United States of America*, *101*(30), 11076–81. doi:10.1073 /pnas.0402970101

Ober, R., Martinez, C., Vaccaro, C., Zhou, J. & Ward, E. (2004). Visualizing the site and dynamics of IgG salvage by the MHC class I-related receptor, FcRn. *Journal of Immunology*, *172*(4), 2021–9.

Pant, N., Hultberg, A., Zhao, Y., Svensson, L., Pan-Hammarstrom, Q Johansen, K., Pouwels, P., … & Hammarstrom, L. (2006). Lactobacilli expressing variable domain of llama heavy-chain antibody fragments (lactobodies) confer protection against rotavirus-induced diarrhea. *Journal of Infectious Diseases*, *194*(11), 1580–8.

Parreño, V., Marcoppido, G., Vega, C., Garaicoechea, L., Rodriguez, D., Saif, L. & Fernández, F. (2010). Milk supplemented with immune colostrum: protection against rotavirus diarrhea and modulatory effect on the systemic and mucosal antibody responses in calves experimentally challenged with bovine rotavirus. *Veterinary Immunology and Immunopathology*, *136*(1-2), 12–27.

Parreño, V., Béjar, C., Vagnozzi, A., Barrandeguy, M., Costantini, V., Craig, M., … & Fernández, F. (2004). Modulation by colostrum-acquired maternal antibodies of systemic and mucosal antibody responses to rotavirus in calves experimentally challenged with bovine rotavirus. *Veterinary Immunology and Immunopathology*, *100*(1-2), 7–24.

Parreño, V., Hodgins, D., DeArriba, L., Kang, S., Yuan, L., Ward, L., … & Saif, L. (1999). Serum and intestinal isotype antibody responses to Wa human rotavirus in gnotobiotic pigs are modulated by maternal antibodies.

The Journal of General Virology, *80 (Pt 6)*, 1417–28. Retrieved from http://www.ncbi.nlm.nih.gov/pubmed/10374959

Quigley, J. 3rd & Drewry, J. (1998). Nutrient and immunity transfer from cow to calf pre- and postcalving. *Journal of Dairy Science*, *81*(10), 2779–90.

Raghavan, M., Bonagura, V., Morrison, S. & Bjorkman, P. (1995). Analysis of the pH dependence of the neonatal Fc receptor/immunoglobulin G interaction using antibody and receptor variants. *Biochemistry*, *34*(45), 14649–57.

Ravetch, J. (1997). Fc receptors. *Current Opionion in Immunology*, *9*, 121–125. doi:10.1016/S0952-7915(97)80168-9

Saif, L. & Fernandez, F. (1996). Group A rotavirus veterinary vaccines. *The Journal of Infectious Diseases*, *174 Suppl*, S98–106. Retrieved from http://www.ncbi.nlm.nih.gov/pubmed/8752298

Salmon, H. (2000). Mammary gland immunology and neonate protection in pigs. Homing of lymphocytes into the MG. *Advances in Experimental Medicine and Biology*, *480*, 279–86.

Salmon, H., Berri, M., Gerdts, V. & Meurens, F. (2009). Humoral and cellular factors of maternal immunity in swine. *Developmental & Comparative Immunology*, *33*(3), 384–93.

Sarker, S., Pant, N., Juneja, L. & Hammarström, L. (2007). Successful treatment of rotavirus-induced diarrhea in suckling mice with egg yolk immunoglobulin. *Journal of Health, Population, and Nutrition*, *25*(4), 465–8.

Schade, R., Calzado, E., Sarmiento, R., Chacana, P., Porankiewicz-Asplund, J. & Terzolo, H. (2005). Chicken egg yolk antibodies (IgY-technology): a review of progress in production and use in research and human and veterinary medicine. *Alternatives to Laboratory Animals: ATLA*, *33*(2), 129–54.

Sfeir, R., Dubarry, M., Boyaka, P., Rautureau, M. & Tomé, D. (2004). The mode of oral bovine lactoferrin administration influences mucosal and systemic immune responses in mice. *The Journal of Nutrition*, *134*(2), 403–9. Retrieved from http://www.ncbi.nlm.nih.gov/pubmed/14747680

Sidell, N., RamaRao, G., Tompkins, W. & Hansen, L. (1979). Phagocytic and Fc receptor functions of alveolar macrophages in cats following ingestion of hexachlorobenzene. *Veterinary and Human Toxicology*, *21*(4), 254–7.

Stelwagen, K., Carpenter, E., Haigh, B., Hodgkinson, a.& Wheeler, T. T. (2009). Immune components of bovine colostrum and milk. *Journal of Animal Science*, *87*(13 Suppl), 3–9. doi:10.2527/jas.2008-1377

Tesar, D., Cheung, E. & Bjorkman, P. (2008). The Chicken Yolk Sac IgY Receptor, a Mammalian Mannose Receptor Family Member, Transcytoses IgY across Polarized Epithelial Cells. *Molecular Biology of the Cell*, *19*(April), 1587–1593. doi:10.1091/mbc.E07

Tini, M., Jewell, U., Camenisch, G., Chilov, D. & Gassmann, M. (2002). Generation and application of chicken egg-yolk antibodies. *Omparative Biochemistry and Physiology. Part A, Molecular & Integrative Physiology*, *131*(3), 569–74.

Trowald-Wigh, G., Ohannisson, A. & Håkansson, L. (1993). Canine neutrophil adhesion proteins and Fc-receptors in healthy dogs and dogs with adhesion protein deficiency, as studied by flow cytometry. *Veterinary Immunology and Immunopathology*, *38*(3-4), 297310.

Tuboly, S. & Bernáth, S. (2002). Intestinal absorption of colostral lymphoid cells in newborn animals. *Advances in Experimental Medicine and Biology*, *503*, 107–14.

Van Hooijdonk, A., Kussendrager, K. & Steijns, J. (2000). In vivo antimicrobial and antiviral activity of components in bovine milk and colostrum involved in non-specific defense. *British Journal of Nutrition*, *84*(1), 127–34.

Vanlandschoot, P., Stortelers, C., Beirnaert, E., Ibañez, L., Schepens, B., Depla, E. & Saelens, X. (2011). Nanobodies®: new ammunition to battle viruses. *Antiviral Research*, *92*(3), 389–407.

Vaughn, D. & Bjorkman, P. (1998). Structural basis of pH-dependent antibody binding by the neonatal Fc receptor. *Structure*, *6*(1), 63–73.

Vega, C., Bok, M., Chacana, P., Saif, L., Fernandez, F. & Parreño, V. (2011). Egg yolk IgY: Protection against rotavirus induced diarrhea and modulatory effect on the systemic and mucosal antibody responses in newborn calves. *Veterinary Immunology and Immunopathology*, *142*, 156–169.

Vega, C., Bok, M., Vlasova, A., Chattha, K., Gomez-Sebastian, S., Nuñez, C., ... & Parreño, V. (2013). Recombinant Monovalent Llama-Derived Antibody Fragments (VHH) to Rotavirus VP6 Protect Neonatal Gnotobiotic Piglets against Human Rotavirus-Induced Diarrhea. *Plos Pathogens*, *9*(5). Retrieved from http://www.plospathogens.org/article/info:doi/10.1371/journal.ppat.1003334

Vega, C. G., Bok, M., Vlasova, A. N., Chattha, K. S., Fernández, F. M., Wigdorovitz, A., ... & Saif, L. J. (2012). IgY antibodies protect against human Rotavirus induced diarrhea in the neonatal gnotobiotic piglet disease model. *PlosOne*, *7*(8). Retrieved from http://www.plosone.org/article/info:doi/10.1371/journal.pone.0042788

Waldmann, T. & Strober, W. (1969). Methabolism of immunoglobulins. *Progress in Allergy*, *13*, 1–110.

Waldner, C. & Rosengren, L. (2009). associated with serum immunoglobulin levels in beef calves from Alberta and Saskatchewan and association between passive transfer and health outcomes. *The Canadian Veterinary Journal*, (7), 275–281. Retrieved from http://www.ncbi.nlm.nih.gov/pmc/articles/PMC2643452/

West, A., Herr, A. & Bjorkman, P. (2004). The Chicken Yolk Sac IgY Receptor, a Functional Equivalent of the Mammalian MHC-Related Fc Receptor, Is a Phospholipase A 2 Receptor Homolog The crystal structures of the ectodomains of rat FcRn. *Immunity*, *20*, 601–610.

Xu, R., Wang, F. & Zhang, S. (2000). Postnatal adaptation of the gastrointestinal tract in neonatal pigs: a possible role of milk-borne growth factors. *Livestock Production Science*, *66*(2), 95–107. doi:10.1016/S0301-6226(00)00217-7

Xu, Y., Li, X., Jin, L., Zhen, Y., Lu, Y., Li, S., ... & Wang, L. (2011). Application of chicken egg yolk immunoglobulins in the control of terrestrial and aquatic animal diseases: a review. *Biotechnology Advances*, *29*(6), 860–8.

Xu, Y., Zou, W., Zhan, X., Yang, S., Xie, D. & Peng, S. (2006). Preparation and determination of immunological activities of anti-HBV egg yolk extraction. *Cellular & Molecular Immunology*, *3*(1), 67–71. Retrieved from http://www.ncbi.nlm.nih.gov/pubmed/16549053

Yamanaka, H., Hagiwara, K., Kirisawa, R. & Iwai, H. (2003). Proinflammatory cytokines in bovine colostrum potentiate the mitogenic response of peripheral blood mononuclear cells from newborn calves through IL-2 and CD25 expression. *Microbial Immunology*, *47*(6), 461–8.

In: Rotavirus Infections
Editor: Carissa D. Zeni
ISBN: 978-1-63321-442-2

Chapter 5

Epidemiology of Rotavirus Infection in Cattle, Small Ruminants and Horses

***Alejandra Badaracco*[1], *Lorena Garaicoeachea*[1], *Jelle Mathijnssens*[2] *and Viviana Parreño*[1,*]**
[1]Instituto de Virologia, CICV y A INTA, Castelar, Argentina
[2]Laboratory of Clinical and Epidemiological Virology, Rega Institute for Medical Research, University of Leuven, Leuven, Belgium

Abstract

Group A Rotavirus (RVA)isa naked virus belonging to the *Reoviridae* family. The virus genome is composed of 11 segments of double stranded RNA. Rotavirus diarrhea is a high morbidity syndrome affecting the young of a large number of animal species. Rotavirus is the main cause of neonatal diarrhea in calves and foals in Argentina and worldwide, strains affecting these two species showed distinct genome constellations. Rotavirus circulation has also been reported in small ruminants as sheep and goats as well as in wild and domestics South American Camelids (llamas, alapacas, guanacos and vicugnas) and old world camelids (Dromedary and Bactrian camelids). The genome analysis of the RVA strain infecting these animal species revealed the

* E-mail: parreno.viviana@inta.gob.ar.

presence of a genome constellation specific of the mammalian order Artiodactyla. The present review summarized the results obtained by our group research over the last twenty years regarding the epidemiology and molecular characterization of RVA circulating in different animal species of economic interest from Argentina, compared with the finding in these species reported worldwide.

Introduction

Group A Rotavirus (RVA) is a naked virus belonging to the *Reoviridae* family. Rotavirus diarrhea is a high morbidity syndrome affecting the young of a large number of animal species. It represents the main cause of neonatal diarrhea in calves and foals, worldwide [1, 2]. Rotavirus circulation has also been reported in small ruminant such as sheep and goats as well as in wild and domestics South American Camelids (llamas, alpacas, guanacos and vicugnas) and Old World Camelids (Dromedary and Bactrian camelids), all species belonging to the order *Artilodactyla* [3-8]. Rotavirus virions are characterized by non-enveloped triple-layered viral particles with a genome composed of 11 double-stranded RNA segments (dsRNA).Each segment codifies for one viral structural (VP1 to VP6)or nonstructural protein (NSP1 to NSP5), except for segment 11, which possesses a second open-reading frame (ORF) in some RVA strains leading to the expression of another non-structural protein (NSP6)in addition to NSP5 [9].

The variability of a group antigen present in the inner capsid protein VP6 allows the classification of rotavirus in 7 serological species or groups (A-G) [10]. Group A rotaviruses are widely distributed infecting human infants and the young of a large variety of animal species [9]. Based on the genetic and antigenic variation of the two outer capsid proteins VP7 (surface Glycoprotein) and VP4 (Protease sensitive spike protein), Group A rotaviruses (RVA) are further classified into G and P types, respectively. These two outer capsid proteins also induce neutralizing antibodies in the infected animals, which are associated with protecting the infection and disease [11].

In April 2008, a Rotavirus Classification Working Group (RCWG) was formed and a nucleotide sequence-based, complete genome classification system was developed for the harmonization of RVA taxonomy. This system assigns a specific genotype to each of the 11 genome segments of a particular RVA strain, according to established nucleotide percent cut-off values. Using this approach, the genome of individual RVA strains are given the complete descriptor of Gx-P [x]-Ix-Rx-Cx-Mx-Ax-Nx-Tx-Ex-Hx assigned as a genome constellation [12, 13]. In the present chapter, we summarized the results obtained by our group of research over the last twenty years regarding the epidemiology and molecular characterization of RVA circulating in calves, foals, guanacos, vicugnas and goat from Argentina, compared with the finding in these species reported worldwide. The genome analysis of the RVA strain infecting these animal species revealed the presence of a genome constellation specific of the mammalian order *Artiodactyla* [14, 15].

Neonatal Calf Diarrhea and Bovine Rotavirus

Neonatal calf diarrhea represent an important sanitary problem in livestock production, it is a complex syndrome affecting calves within the first 4 weeks of life, causing important economic losses related to death, treatment costs and reduction in weight gain of affected animals. The etiology of the disease involves diverse infectious agents (virus, bacteria and protozoa) and is worsened by several factors including herd management, environment, and host nutritional and immunological conditions [16, 17].

As regards the microbiology, calf diarrhea has been historically attributed to bovine rotavirus group A (BRV-A), bovine coronavirus (BCoV), *Salmonella spp.*, enteropathogenic strains of *Escherichia coli* carrying intestinal and extra-intestinal virulent factors, *Clostridium perfringens* and *Cryptosporidium parvum* [18].Usually the diarrhea is caused by a combination of these agents, however the specific etiology of many field cases of calf diarrhea still remain undiagnosed, suggesting that other agents are involved in this disease. Rotavirus group B and C were also reported to infect cattle but their impact associated to neonatal calf diarrhea remains unknown. To date, RVB were found in adult cattle or calves with diarrhea from India, Japan and USA [19-22], while rotavirus C was recently reported to be present in seven out of 127 (5.5%) calves with diarrhea from 52 herds (13.5%) surveyed in South Korea. Interestingly, the study found strains belonging to the bovine lineage and also strains belonging to the porcine lineage that can infect and cause diarrhea in calves [23].

In the 2000 decade, bovine norovirus (BNoV, Nebovirus, bovine enterovirus (BEV) and bovine torovirus (BToV)were identified as potential causes of calf diarrhea) [24, 25].A case control study conducted in dairy farms from the Midwest USA demonstrated that BNoV (OR = 2.0) and Nebovirus (OR = 16.7) had a significant contribution to calf diarrhea [24]. Cho and co-workers (2013) reported that calves shedding 2 or more pathogens were 6 times more likely to develop clinical diarrhea compared with the ones that shed only one or no pathogen [24]. They also studied how the presence of one pathogen can increase the incidence of another one. For example, the presence of Rotavirus increased 2.2-fold the odds of detecting *Cryptosporidium parvum* [24].

Regarding management, calf diarrhea is a disease that could be avoided by good management practices, yet it is the most common cause of death in young calves. Most fatal diarrhea occurs in the first two weeks after birth. As calves grow older, their susceptibility to infections decreases rapidly but remains significant until three to four weeks of age. Since the multifactor pathology of calf diarrhea prevention should be considered globally within the farm. Two factors have been demonstrated to be beneficial to decrease the risk of disease in a herd: i) herd hygiene and ii) dam vaccination [16, 26].In general, dam vaccination against at least one of the major infectious agents late in gestation decreased the risk of diarrhea. Calves born to a non-vaccinated herd had a 2.1 times higher risk of diarrhea than calves born to vaccinated dams [16].

In Argentina, 5% of the newborn calves die before weaning, mainly due to diarrhea and respiratory syndromes [27]. Surveys conducted in beef and dairy herds from 1994 to 2010covering five ecological regions (Humid and DryPampa, Mesopotamia, Patagonia and Cuyo) indicated that bovine RVA is broadly distributed, being detected in all the regions and participating in55% of the diarrhea outbreaks studied [1, 28] (Figure 1). A similar survey was conducted in Brazil covering several states from four geographical regions [29]. Bovine RVA was detected in all the regions analyzed, however the incidence of RVA diarrhea in terms of positive samples was lower (19.4%) compared with the incidence found in Argentina (36%) (Figure 1). These differences could be related to differential weather, husbandry systems, rearing conditions and the biotype of cattle breed in each country. Regarding the incidence of RVA diarrhea and the type of husbandry, in Argentina, the detection rate of RVA was significantly higher in beef (64%; 216/336)than in dairy herds (54 %; 103/191), Chi square, p=0.0193. However, these incidences, both higher than 50%, indicate that RVA represents an important pathogen contributing to calf diarrhea [1, 28].

A systematic review conducted by Papp, et. al (2013) including 75 articles published during the past 30 years including surveys conducted in 24 countries from the 5 continents found that RVA was detected in 33.7% (4749/14,076) of the bovine samples tested, demonstrating its extent of distribution and incidence in cattle livestock, worldwide [30].

YEARS	Total outbreaks (samples)	RVA detection rate (% outbreaks)	RVA detection rate (% samples)
1994-2010	823 (3043)	55% (455/823)	36% (1098/3043)

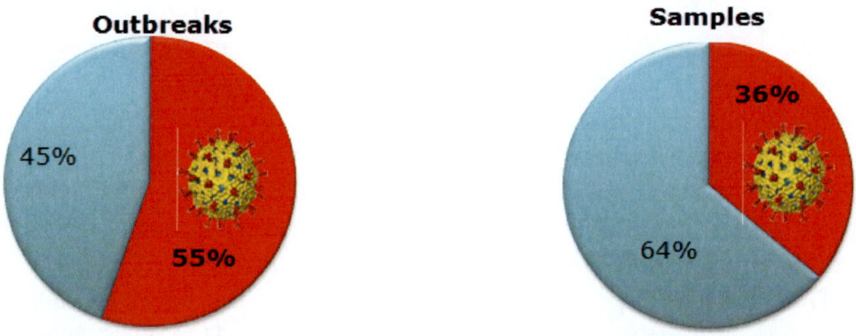

Summarized from Garaicoechea L., et. al. Veterinary Microbiology 118 (2006) 1–11 and Badaracco, A. et al. Vet. Microbiology, 58 (2012), 394-399 and Badaracco, PhD, thesis, 2011.

Figure 1. Rotavirus detection rate in calves with diarrhea.

The results summarized in that study places important questions regarding vaccine application, coverage and efficacy.

Rotavirus Strains Circulating in Cattle

Rotavirus strains are classified into G and P-types based on the genetic and antigenic variation of the two outer capsid proteins VP7 and VP4, respectively [9, 31]. To date, 27 G types and 37 P types have been recognized [12, 32, 33].Numerous RVA genotypes have been detected in calves, with at least 12 different G types (G1-G3, G6, G8,G10, G11, G15, G17, G21 and G24) and 11 different P types (P [1], P [3], P [5], P [6], P [7], P [11], P [14], P [17], P [21], P [29]and P [33]) reported [1, 28, 33-39] G6, G8,G10 associated to P [5], P [11] and, to a lesser extent with P [1] are considered epidemiologically important in cattle [30]. The conducted surveys have shown that the prevalent RVAstrains circulating in Argentinean cattle belong to the typical bovine genotypes G6, G10, P [5] and P [11] [1, 15, 28, 40]. These results are in concordance with the global bovine RVA epidemiology. Papp et. al. (2013) found that G6 is the prevalent G-type (56.7%) followed by G10 (20.6%), while G8 is circulating in bovines, but at a much lower rate (3.5%).The predominant P-types circulating in cattle worldwide are P [5]and P [11] both with similar detection rates, 25.6% and 21.5%, respectively [30]. This systematic review also showed that there is a high amount of untypable samples, especially for P-typing (43.6%) [30], which could indicate the circulation of a new strain or a failure of the typing techniques.

Regarding geographical distribution G6 strains are present in the 5 continents, G10 was found in America, Europe, Asia and Australia, while G8 is mostly found in Africa. Both P [5] and P [11] are circulating in cattle from all continents except Africa [30](Figure 2).

Three G and P combinations, G6P [5], G6P [11] and G10P [11], were prevalent representing 40.4% of the overall circulating strains. An interesting finding observed in Argentinean surveys was that there is a clear differential distribution of G and P types depending on herd husbandry.

Thus, G6(IV)P [5] strains were most prevalent in beef herds, while similar proportions of G6(III)P [11], G6(IV)P [11] and G10P [11] were detected in dairy herds [1, 15, 28, 40] (Figure 3; Table 1).

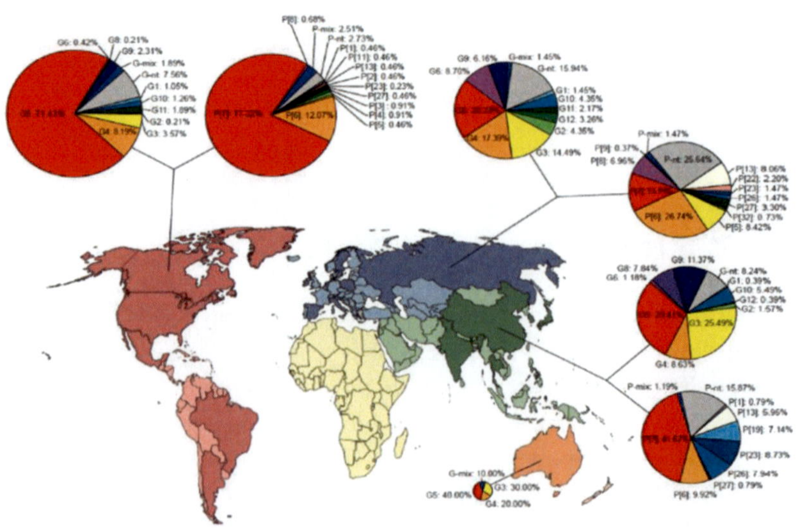

Figure 2. RVA G and P distribution in cattle, worldwide. Extracted from Papp, 2013.

The differential epidemiology for the distribution of G and P types according to the exploitation type was maintained over time, and is more marked for the P type than the G types, with P [5] being the most prevalent genotype in beef herds and P [11] is the most prevalent in dairy herds. This finding is not easy to explain but it could be speculated that this is the effect of different rearing conditions of beef and dairy calves. In beef herds under extensive management, the calving season is scheduled once a year, resulting in a long period without newborns. The G6(IV)P [5] RVA strains may be more resistant to the environment, or they may circulate asymptomatically for longer period in the adult cattle population. The yearly bottleneck without susceptible newborns could explain the lower genetic RVA diversity observed in beef herds. Conversely, in dairy farms calves are born all year around and reared under artificial conditions hence there are always susceptible hosts, allowing fora larger variety of different G/P-genotypes to co-circulate in dairy herds, even those of low virulence.

Another important behavior of RVA infection in cattle is the high percentages of co-infections and co-circulation of bovine RVA strains with different genotypes registered in both exploitation systems (20%in beef and 23% in dairy).Co-circulation was considered when in the same outbreak there were different calves shedding a distinct bovine RVA straining each one; farms with co-circulation also included calves shedding a unique strain together with calves suffering aco-infection. This finding are also reported in other countries, in fact a systematic review including surveys conducted in the 5 continents reported that mixed infections are detected in 5.9% for G types and 6.2% for P types of the tested samples (14,076) [30]. Mixed infections represent the main mechanism of RVA diversity, leading to genetic reassortment.

Phylogenetic Analyses of Typical Bovine Rotavirus Genotypes G6, G10,P [5] and P [11]

The phylogeny is the study of the evolutive relationships. The molecular information such like amino acid and nucleotidic sequences are used to investigate the evolution and the phylogenetic relationship between the different bovine RVA strains.

Basically, the phylogenetic methods compare the similarity of homologous genes or segments, inferring the common history between them, using a tree.

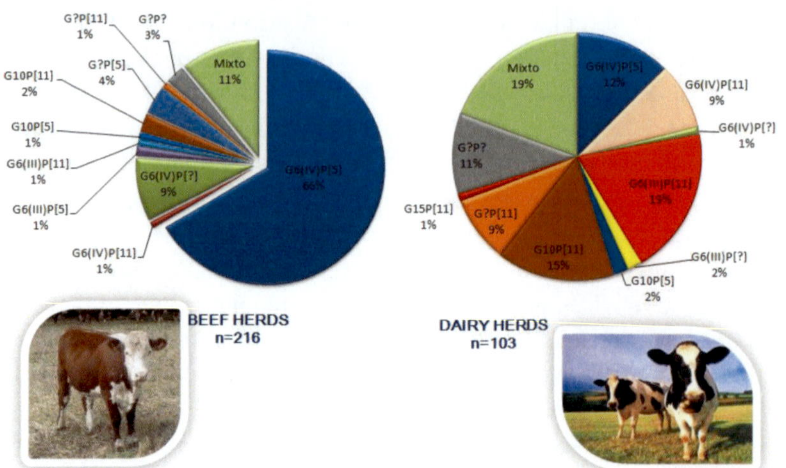

Summarized from Garaicoechea L., et al. Veterinary Microbiology 118 (2006) 1–11 and Badaracco, A. et al. Vet. Microbiology, 58 (2012), 394-399 and Badaracco, PhD, thesis, 2011.

Figure 3. Bovine Rotavirus: Circulating genotypes in beef and dairy herds in Argentina (1994-2010).

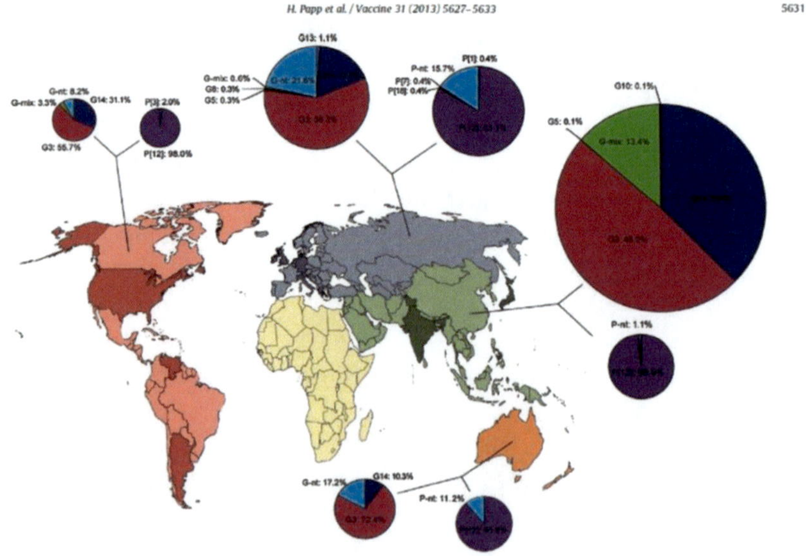

Figure 4.Global distribution of equine RVA.

Table 1. G and P typing of BRV strains circulating in Argentinean calves from 1994 to 2010

Exploitation Type	Surveyed period	Nº of farms													
		G6(IV) P [5]	G6(IV) P [11]	G6(IV) P [?]	G6(III) P [5]	G6(III) P [11]	G6(III) P [?]	G10 P [5]	G10 P [11]	G10 P [?]	G? P [5]	G? P [11]	G?P?	Mixed	Total
Beef	1994-2003	114	1	8	3			2	3		5	1	5	10	152
	2004-2010	39	1	2		2			3		5	1	1	13	67
Subtotal Beef	**1994-2010**	**153**	**2**	**9**	**3**	**2**		**2**	**6**		**9**	**2**	**6**	**25**	**219**
Dairy	1994-2003	4	5	1		10		2	5			6	1	4	38
	2004-2010	9	4			10	2		11			4	10	15	65
Subtotal Dairy		**13**	**9**	**1**		**20**	**2**	**2**	**16**			**9**	**11**	**20**	**103**
Non specified	1994-2003	33	5	4		1	1	2	3	1	2	2	4	4	62
	2004-2010	46	3	2		3		1	3			2	3	12	75
Subtotal		**79**	**8**	**5**		**4**	**1**	**3**	**6**	**1**	**2**	**4**	**4**	**17**	**137**
Non specified															
Total	**1994-2010**	**245**	**19**	**15**	**3**	**26**	**3**	**7**	**28**	**1**	**11**	**15**	**24**	**62**	**459**

[a] Column assigned as "Mixed" included co-infections (calves shedding BRV with nested-PCR products corresponding to more than one G or P types) and Mixed infections (different calves in the same herd shedding a distinct BRV strain in each one).

Summarized from Garaicoechea L., et al., Veterinary Microbiology 118 (2006) 1–11; Badaracco, A. et al., Vet. Microbiology, 58 (2012), 394-399 and Badaracco, PhD, thesis, 2011.

The phylogenetical trees show the evolutive relationship between the genes and the organism. In Virology, the phylogenetical analyses have been very useful for study the different biological pattern of diversity in a historical context and taxonomy studies.

Different methods are used to construct the phylogenetic tree, like Maximum Parsimony, Maximum Likelihood, Bayesian Methods and Distances Methods. The most common used in the phylogenetical RVA analysis are the Distances Methods. Usually, the distances methods use evolutive models that correct the problem of the multiple substitutions.

Here we summarized the phylogenetic analysis of bovine RVA strains belonging to the prevalent genotypes circulating in cattle: G6, G10, P [5] and P [11] [1, 15, 28, 40].Analyses of VP7 data using G6 sequences of the entire world confirmed that the G6 genotype could be divided into 5 lineages [1, 41, 42]. Lineage I is composed of human G6 RVA strains in combination with P [6] and P [9]. Lineage II is formed by human G6P [14] RVA strains from different countries, one G6P [14] RVA strain was detected in an antelope (RC18/08) from South Africa, two RVA strains found in goats (Cap455 from South Africa and GO34from Bangladesh), a bovine strain from India and two porcine strains from India. Lineage III constitutes a monophyletic group and comprises human G6P [9] RVA strains from Hungary, a buffaloG6P [3] from Italy and bovine strains from Hungary and Argentina in combination with P [5] and P [11]. G6 lineage IV comprises typical P [1], P [5] and P [11] bovine RVA strains from all over the world, 3bovine RVA P [7] strains, one equine strain from India and one porcine strain from Argentina [43]. Finally, lineage V includes bovine strains and one human strain from Hungary (Figure 5).

The fact that G6(III) strains are highly prevalent in Argentinean cattle and have been detected in humans, merits the continuous co-surveillance of children with diarrhea living in rural areas together with animal samples, including pets and livestock. Importantly, the five lineages observed at the nucleotide level were also obtained in the phylogenetic tree constructed with deduced amino acid sequences, indicating that many of the mutations in the nucleotide sequences were translated in amino acid changes. The amino acid differences between G6(III) andG6(IV) strains include 7 amino acid substitutions in known antigenic regions. Moreover, the G6 (III) Argentinean strains presented2 glycosylation sites as opposed to the G6 vaccine strains presented3 glycosylation sites, which can have a strong influence on the antigenic properties [1, 15, 28, 40].

These findings suggest that vaccine induced antibodies could have a lower cross-neutralizing activity against strains belonging to different lineages of G6.

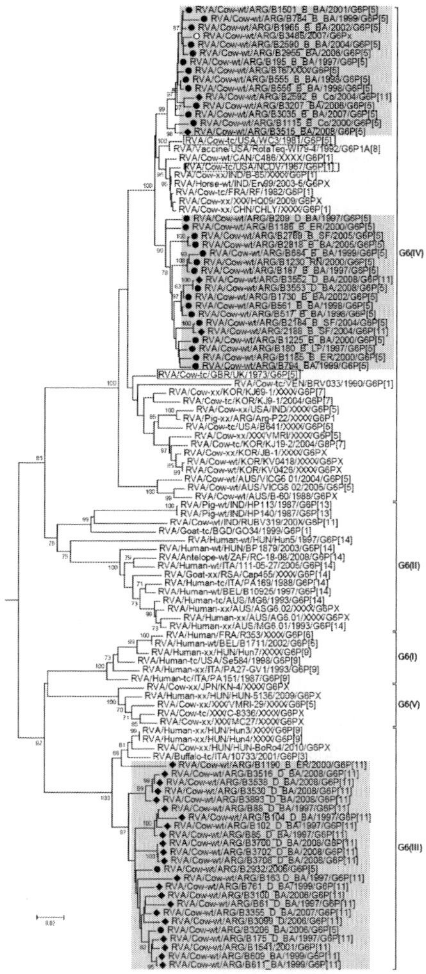

Figure 5. Bioinformatic analyses of G6 genotype. The phylogenetic tree was constructed using the Kimura 2-parameter and Neighbor-Joining methods using the program MEGA5. Bootstrap values are shown at the branch nodes. The lineages are indicated at the right hand side. The Argentinean strains isolated are shown in grey boxes and the vaccines strains are indicated with open squares. In the Argentinean strains: name of the strain, type of exploitation and province of collection are shown. Abbreviations: D/B, Dairy or Beef; BA, Buenos Aires; SF, Santa Fe; Co, Cordoba; RN, Rio Negro; ER, Entre Rios; LP, La Pampa; ♦ G6P [11]; ● G6P [5]; ○ G6Px.

However, in vitro studies have shown cross-neutralization between RVA strains belonging to lineage V (KN4) and lineage IV (NCDV Lincoln) [44]. In addition, protection studies performed ongnotobiotic calves demonstrated that the immunity induced by a bovine RVA strain belonging to G6(V) conferred protection against challenge with a G6(IV) strain [45]. The genetic distances between lineages V and IV (16.7–20.6%) and lineages III and IV (16.2–22%) are very similar suggesting that despite the differences observed at the nucleotide and amino acid level, from the antigenic point of view, cross-neutralization and cross-protection should exist between the two G6 lineages circulating in cattle based on these *in silico* analysis. Further cross neutralization studies are needed to confirm this hypothesis.

G10 is the second most prevalent RVA genotype in cattle. Phylogenetic analyses identified six distinct G10 genotype lineages (Figure 6) [1, 15, 28, 40].

Briefly, lineage I is composed of humanG10 RVA strains from Africa, lineage II includes bovine and equine RVA strains from India and one human RVA strain from Thailand. Lineage III and IV contain only one strain, the human strain RVA/Human-tc/GBR/A64/1987/G10P [11] from England and the sheep strain RVA/Sheep-tc/CHN/Lamb-NT/XXXX/G10P [15] from China, respectively. G10 lineage V is composed of large diversity of strains, including a G10P [11] buffalo RVA strain(RVA/Buffalo-XX/ZAF/Buf1442-07SA/2007/G10P [11]), a G10P [5]porcine RVA strain P343 and bovine strains from all over the world(e.g.: India, Australia, China, USA and Thailand), including the bovine vaccine strain B223 from the USA and one Argentinean strain(RVA/cow-wt/ARG/B3326_D_BA/2007/G10P [11]) from a dairy herd from Buenos Aires.

Of note, this lineage comprises two reassortant human-bovine RVA strains (I321 and N155 G10P [11]) detected in children from India (Bhandari et al., 2006; Ramani et al., 2009).

Finally, lineage VI is composed by Argentinean bovineG10 strains that formed a monophyletic group together with the RVA strain (RVA/Human-xx/BRA/R239/2000-4/G10P [9]) from Brazil(Figure 6) [40, 46].G10 genotype possesses a high potential to infect other animal species including buffaloes, horses, pigs and lambs. The detection of a buffaloG10P [3] RVA strain in India, with a P type closely related to strains isolated from dogs, monkeys and goats, strongly supports the ability of G10 RVA strains to jump the species barrier and reassort [47].

This genotype also possesses a strong zoonotic transmission potential to humans as previously reported [46, 48-50].

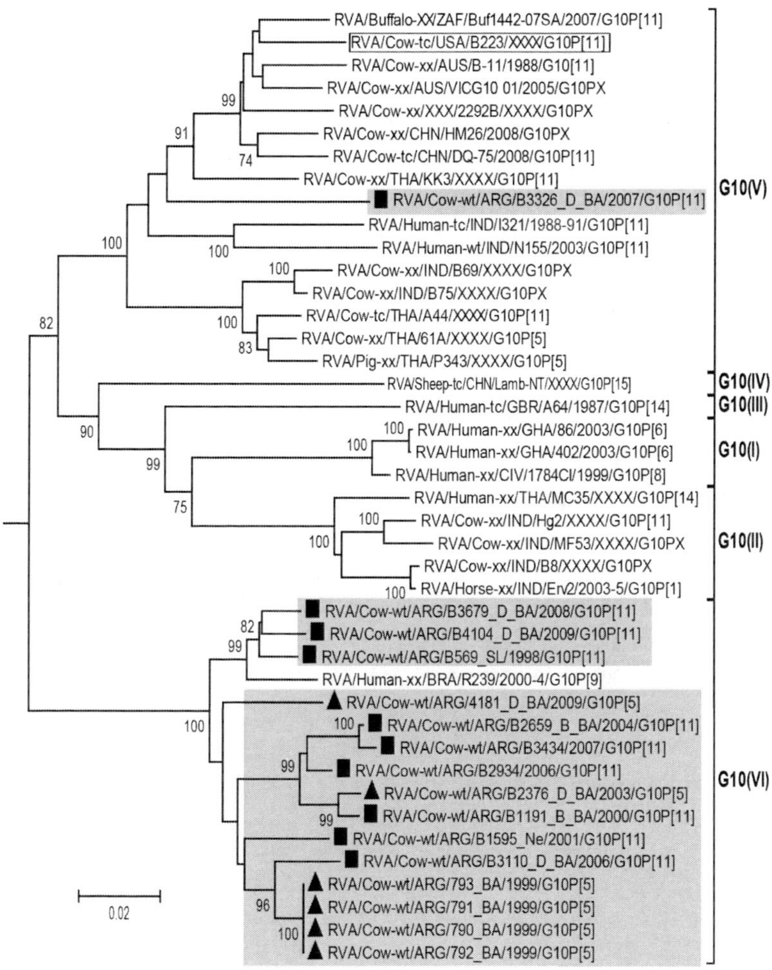

Figure 6. Bioinformatic analyses of G10 genotype. (A) The nucleotide tree was constructed using the Kimura 2-parameter and Neighbor-Joining methods using the program MEGA5. Bootstrap values are shown at the branch nodes. The lineages are indicated at the right hand side. The Argentinean strains isolated are shown in grey boxes and the vaccines strains are indicated with open squares. In the Argentinean strains: name of the strain, type of exploitation and province of collection are shown. Abbreviations: D/B, Dairy or Beef; BA, Buenos Aires; SL, San Luis; Ne, Neuquén; ■ G10P [11]; ▲ G10P [5].

Several G10P [11] bovine-human and G10P [8] human-bovine-porcine reassortant strains have been found in symptomatic and asymptomatic children from India and Hungary, respectively [48-50]. The fact that the Argentinean bovines G10(VI)RVA strains clustered together with an unusual G10P [9] RVA strain detected in 2-year-old hospitalized child with severe diarrhea and dehydration from Rio de Janeiro, during the seasons 2000–2004 [46], reinforces the significant zoonotic potential of G10 RVA strains [40, 46]. The tree constructed with the deduced amino acid sequences showed three lineages supported only by low bootstrap values. These results, together with the direct inspection of the alignments showed that the mutations observed at the nucleotide level were translated only in 4 amino acid changes within the antigenic sites. Thus, although different lineages can be determined using nucleotide data, at the protein level theG10 strains seem to remain rather similar. The low level of amino acid mutations in G10 strains contrast with the amino acid diversity of G6 strains, which could be due to structural constraints presented by the VP7 protein from G10 strains while the one from the G6strains could allow more plasticity.

Lineages were also determined for bovine P-genotypes P [5] and P [11] [40]. The P [5] genotype is characteristic of RVA strains affecting cattle and is broadly distributed all over [1, 28, 35-37, 39, 51]. From the topology of the dendrogram, eight lineages were defined (Figure 7). Lineage I and II were solely composed of bovine Argentinean RVA strains from different provinces and years. Lineage I only included G6(IV)P [5] Argentinean strains belonging to beef herds, while lineage II included G6P [5] and G10P [5] Argentinean strains belonging to both beef and dairy herds. Lineage III was composed of a bovine and a porcine strain from Thailand and one bovine strain from the UK. Lineage IV only possessed the Chinese strain RVA/Pig-xx/CHN/ 4S/XXXX/G3P [5]. Lineage V and VI included the reference strains UK andWC3 respectively. Lineage VII is composed by the RVA strain RVA/Cow-tc/USA/B641/XXXX/G6P7 [5]. Finally, Lineage VIII is formed by 3 bovine strains from the UK, USA and Korea, one human strain from the USA and the strain WI 79-9 included in the human vaccine Rotateq [40]. The strong association of the P [5] genotype with G6(IV) is remarkable. Thus, out of the 12 of P [5] described in the literature, only three RVA carrying P [5] genotype were detected either in other species or associated to other genotypes: the strains P343 (G10P [5]) and 4S (G3P [5]) were detected in pigs from Thailand and China, respectively; and the human strain CJN-M (G1P [5]) was detected in the United States [52].The phylogenetic analyses using different approaches indicated that the P [5] genotype can be divided into eight lineages. Although, lineages I and II were only composed of Argentinean strains that were rather similar to each other (4.2–6.4%), and the other six lineages contained more divergent strains. It's important to highlight that, at the amino acid level, the field strains were distantly related to the strain included in the vaccine formulations used to prevent calf diarrhea (Lineage I vs. Lineage V, 3.2–6.9%; Lineage II vs. Lineage V, 3.6–7.2% amino acid genetic distance).

Phylogenetic analyses of P [11] VP8* revealed that this type can be divided into six lineages at the nucleotide level. The analyses conducted with amino acid sequences confirmed the presence of three phylogenetic lineages among the P [11] strains. All Argentinean strains clustered within lineage III with other strains detected worldwide, with no association between lineages and G type, exploitation type, year or location (Figure 7) [40].Genotype P [11] has been found in our surveys and elsewhere in combination with multiple G types (G6, G8, G9 and G15) (Badaracco et al., 2011; Garaicoechea et al., 2006; Ghosh et al., 2008; Matthijnssens et al., 2009). Interestingly, P [11](III) strains have been detected in human samples (Bhandari et al., 2006; Ramani et al., 2009), which highlights the potential interspecies transmission of strains bearing this P type. In contrast to other countries that showed little diversity (Cashman et al., 2010), Argentinean bovine strains showed a large genetic diversity and multiple new clusters tightly related among them and distant from the bovine RVA circulating all over the world. These clusters included strains circulating for over 12 years in the Argentinean cattle. Overall, this could be explained by the different cattle breeds present in Argentina, the two different husbandry system studies, the difference among the ecological areas sampled and the virus biology.

Overall, the phylogenetic study describes the variability within the prevalent genotypes of the bovine RVA strains circulating in the cattle, and studied their relationship with vaccines and other strains circulating worldwide and set the need for further studies to evaluate their zoonotic potential.

These epidemiological surveys and phylogenetic studies are important for the rational design of rotavirus vaccines. A large variety of killed vaccines, parenterally applied to the pregnant cows in last stage of gestation, has been developed and are available in the market. Live attenuated vaccines for calves are also available but only in countries where live vaccination is allowed by their animal health authorities [11]. Vaccination against neonatal calf diarrhea is not mandatory, and little is reported regarding vaccine application and efficacy. Farmers do not necessarily apply the vaccine routinely, but in Argentina, our experience shows that systematic vaccination in every calving season reduces the incidence of RVA diarrhea in beef herds (Parreño, unpublished data).

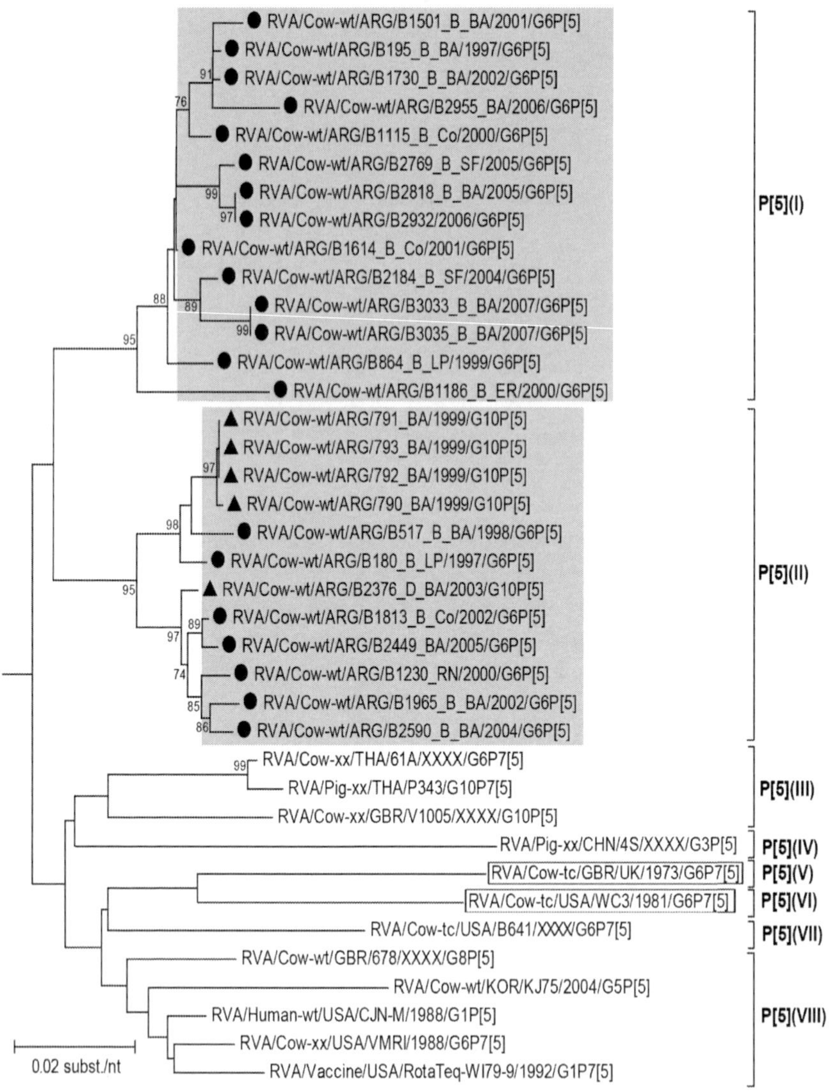

Figure 7.Bioinformatic analyses of the P [5] genotype. (A) The nucleotide tree was constructed using the Kimura 2-parameter and Neighbor-Joining methods using the program MEGA5. Bootstrap values are shown at the branch nodes. The lineages are indicated at the right hand side. The Argentinean strains isolated are shown in grey boxes and the vaccines strains are indicated with open squares. In the Argentinean strains: name of the strain, type of exploitation and province of collection are shown. Abbreviations: D/B, Dairy or Beef; BA, Buenos Aires; SF, Santa Fe; Co, Cordoba; RN, Rio Negro; ER, Entre Rios; LP, La Pampa; • G6P [5]; ▲ G10P [5].

On the other hand, several factors contribute to vaccine failure including inadequate managing conditions, poor vaccine immunogenicity and antigenic differences between the vaccine and field RVA strains [11].

Regarding vaccine quality, the animal health authorities of Argentina have recently adopted a guinea pig model as an alternative method for RVA vaccine potency testing. This official test guarantees the quality of the RVA vaccines that are released to the local market (resol. SENASA 598-12, http://www.cac.com.ar/documentos/17_Res.%20SENASA%20598-12.pdf). Regarding the G and P types covered by the current vaccines, systematic surveys of the genotypes circulating in cattle are very important for vaccine update.

Beside vaccines, other therapeutic tools are under progress, and will be reviewed in another chapter of this book.

Finally, despite the efforts carried out in prevention, the results of the surveys conducted in the last 3 decades demonstrate that rotavirus still represents major cause of calf diarrhea and a sanitary problem of high impact in the livestock industry in Argentina and worldwide.

Complete Genome Studies of Bovine Group A Rotavirus

Whole genome studies of representative strains G6(IV)P [5] prevalent in beef herds, G6(III)P [11] and G10P [11] prevalent in dairy herds (*Badaracco, Ph Thesis, manuscript in preparation*) and the rare strains G8P [11] andG15P [11] found only in one opportunity each, in dairy calves with diarrhea, were conducted and compared with the available constellation of bovines RVA sequenced in America, Europe, Asia and wild species as Buffalo and antelopes from South Africa (Table 2).

All the sequenced strains possess typical bovine G/P-genotype combinations except for the Korean strains carrying a P [7] genotype typically from porcine [53] and the new strains detected in India AzuK-1 (G21P [29]) isolated from an asymptomatic calf and Dai-10 strain, sharing G24P [33] genotypes, previously reported in an asymptomatic cow in Hyogo Prefecture, Japan in 2007 [34].

In recent years it has become clear that RVA strains with similar genotype constellations are also present in other member's species of the family of Artiodactyls such as, vicunas, sheep and antelope and buffaloes [4, 15, 54, 55]. Reassortment events are also very common in the RVA infecting bovines.

Table 2. Gene constellation of Bovine RVA strains

Strain Name	VP7	VP4	VP6	VP1	VP2	VP3	NSP1	NSP2	NSP3	NSP4	NSP5
RVA/cow-wt/ARG/B4385/2011/G8P [11]	G8	P [11]	I2	R5	C2	M2	A13	N2	T6	E12	H3
RVA/cow-wt/ARG/B4104/2009/G6P [5]	G6	P [5]	I2	R5	C2	M2	A3	N2	T6	E12	H3
RVA/cow-wt/ARG/B4104/2009/G10P [11]	G10	P [11]	I2	R5	C2	M2	A13	N2	T6	E12	H3
RVA/cow-wt/ARG/B3700/2008/G6P [11]	G6	P [11]	I2	R5	C2	M2	A3	N2	T6	E12	H3
RVA/Cow-wt/ARG/B383/1998/G15P [11]	G15	P [11]	I2	R5	C2	M2	A13	N2	T6	E12	H3
RVA/Cow-tc/CHN/DQ-75/2008/G10P [11]	G10	P [11]	I2	R2	C2	M2	A3	N2	T6	E2	H3
RVA/Cow-tc/JPN/Dai-10/2007/G24P [33]	G24	P [33]	I2	R2	C2	M2	A13	N2	T9	E2	H3
RVA/Cow-wt/JPN/Azuk-1/2006/G21P [29]	G21	P [29]	I2	R2	C2	M2	A13	N2	T9	E2	H3
RVA/Cow-wt/ZAF/1603-1605/2007/G6P [5]	G6	P [5]	I2	R2	C2	M2		N2	T6	E2	H3
RVA/Cow-wt/ZAF/1604/2007/G8P [1]	G8	P [1]	I2	R2	C2	M2	A3	N2	T6	E2	H3
RVA/Cow-tc/KOR/KJ19-2 2c/2004/G6P [7]	G6	P [7]	I2	R2	C2	M2	A3	N2	T6	E2	H3
RVA/Cow-tc/KOR/KJ9-1 1/2004/G6P [7]	G6	P [7]	I2	R2	C1	M2	A1	N2	T1	E2	H1
RVA/Cow-tc/KOR/KJ25-1/2004/G8P [7]	G8	P [7]	I5	R1	C1	M2	A1	N1	T1	E1	H1
RVA/Cow-tc/JPN/Sun9/2000/G8P [14]	G8	P [14]	I2	R2	C2	M2				E2	

Strain Name	VP7	VP4	VP6	VP1	VP2	VP3	NSP1	NSP2	NSP3	NSP4	NSP5
Strain Name	VP7	VP4	VP6	VP1	VP2	VP3	NSP1	NSP2	NSP3	NSP4	NSP5
RVA/Cow-tc/VEN/BRV033/1990/G6P6 [1]	G6	P [1]	I2	R2	C2	M2	A3	N2	T6	E2	H3
RVA/Cow-tc/FRA/RF/1982/G6P [1]	G6	P [1]	I2	R2	C2	M2	A3	N2	T6	E2	H3
RVA/Cow-tc/USA/WC3/1981/G6P [5]	G6	P [5]	I2	R2	C2	M2	A3	N2	T6	E2	H3
RVA/Cow-tc/GBR/UK/1973/G6P [5]	G6	P [5]	I2	R2	C2	M2	A3	N2	T7	E2	H3
RVA/Cow-tc/USA/NCDV/1967/G6P [1]	G6	P [1]	I2	R2	C2	M2		N2	T6	E2	
RVA/Cow-tc/USA/B223/XXXX/G10P [11]	G10	P [11]	I2				A13			E2	
RVA/Giraffe-wt/IRL/GirRV/2008/G10P [11]	G10	P [11]	I2	R2	C2	M2	A3	N2	T6	E2	H3
RVA/Antelope-wt/ZAF/RC-18/2008/G6P [14]	G6	P [14]	I2	R2	C2	M2	A11	N2	T6	E2	H3
RVA/Buffalo-XX/ZAF/Buf1442-07SA/2007/G10P [11]	G10	P [11]	I2	R2	C2	M2	A13	N2	T6	E2	H3

As examples, phylogenetic analyses showed that VP6 and NSP2 gene segments of the AzuK-1 and Dai-10 strains from Japan were clustered with those of simian or canine/feline rotaviruses, rather than with those of bovine rotaviruses [34]. Park et al. (2011) also reported similar reassortant events of bovine strains carrying porcine and feline/canine genes [53]. RVA with a typical bovine genome constellation was also reported to infect giraffes [56]; reinforcing the statement that the strains circulating in cattle might infect other animal species of the order *Artilodactyla* or that all the viruses infecting these species are genetically related. In addition, this genotype constellation has occasionally been found in other host species including primates (simian and humans) [30, 41, 57] most likely representing individual interspecies transmissions but strongly indicating the zoonotic potential of these RVA strains [31].Regarding the bovine Argentinean RVA strains, all strains possess genotypes typically found in bovine RVA strains except for the VP1 (R5) and NSP4 (E12) that are characteristic of RVA from Argentina [1, 2, 28]. However, the apparent ubiquitous presence of the R5 and E12 genotypes in all analyzed Argentinean bovine RVA strains is intriguing as these genotypes have only been described from South-American samples collected from different species such as cattle, alpacas, horses and guanacos [2, 15, 58], and on one occasion in Brazil from a human child [46].

In conclusion, these data suggest that although a rather conserved bovine RVA genotype constellation was found among different circulating bovine RVA strains, inside these genotypes, there is a wide range of genetically distinct RVA variants. In addition, bovine RVA strains may readily exchange gene segments with other small ruminant and larger members of the family of *Artiodactyla*. Animal-to-human interspecies transmission is one of the evolutionary mechanisms driving rotavirus strain diversity in humans.

Recent whole genome data of African bovine RVA strains genotyped as G6/8-P [5/1]-I2-R2-C2-M2-A3-N2-T6-E2-H3 suggested that these bovine RVA strains may have emerged through multiple reassortment events between bovine, giraffe and antelope rotaviruses. In addition, the close relatedness of some genome segments to those of the corresponding segments of human RVA strains give another example of the transmission to humans [59].

Equine Rotavirus

Since the initial detection of group A equine rotavirus (RVA) in diarrheic foals in England in 1975 [60], it has been detected in outbreaks of neonatal diarrhea in foals in every country with an equine industry [2, 61, 62]. Equine RVA is considered to be the major cause of dehydrating diarrhea in foals younger than 3 month old [63]. Young foals are highly susceptible to RVA infection and develop malabsorptive watery diarrhea leading to severe dehydration and sometimes death, especially in neonates with failure of passive antibody transference. RVA infections very common in horses and all adult populations seropositive for antibodies [64]. In Argentina, ERV associated with diarrhea in foals was first described in 1985 (Valle et al., 1990). Our group of research has been studying equine RVA since 1992. The outbreaks of diarrhea due to equine RVA in thoroughbred breeding farms occur every foaling season during the months of September–October, in concordance with the highest density of susceptible animals. In some horse farms, the outbreaks may affect up to 100% of foals. In the study conducted by Garaicoechea, et al. (2011) equine RVA was detected in 39% of the diarrhea outbreaks registered in 35 thoroughbred horse farms during a 17-year surveillance period (1992–2008), confirming a high incidence of rotavirus disease in thoroughbred horses from Argentina.

Regarding the epidemiology of the disease, the characterized Argentinean strains were shown to belong to genotypes G3 (51%) or G14 (33%); no other G type was detected.

In addition, 4% represented mixed infections with G3 and G14 strains, while 11% of the samples were unable to be typed [2]. G3 equine RVA are further subclassified into two subtypes, G3A and G3B. The Argentinean G3strains were shown to belong to the G3A.

The VP4 of all the Argentinean RVA belonged to the P [12] genotype, except for one G3 equine RVRVA/Horse-wt/ARG/E3198/2008/G3P [3], detected in a horse farm from Buenos Aires province, in 2008, whose VP4 type was P [3] [2].

A recent systematic review of the literature including surveys of equine RVA in diarrheic foals from Europe, America, Asia and Australia demonstrated that over 99% of the equine RVA typed in the last 30 years belonged to two common genotypes: G3P [12] and G14P [12] [62]. The G-genotype G3 was found in 51.7% of the infections while G14 was reported in 32% of the cases. Regarding the G3 subtypes, G3A has been detected in foals from Argentina and also from England (Isa et al., 1996), Ireland (Collins et al., 2008), Australia (Browning and Begg, 1996) United States (Browning et al., 1992a) and Germany (Elschner et al., 2005), while the G3B subtype has been detected in Japan (Tsunemitsu et al., 2001) and United States (Browning et al., 1992a).

Strains belonging to other G-types (G5, G6, G8, G10, G13)and 4 P-types (P [1], P [3], P [7], P [11], and P [18]) have been detected among horses in particular cases, such as RVA G13P [18] L338 strain [65], the porcine-like G5P [7] H-1 strain [66], the bovine-like Eq/26/94 G8P [1] [67] and Eq/R-22 G10P [11] [68] strains and a feline-like G3P [3] strain from Argentina (E3198/Arg/2008) [69]. However these strains did not spread in the equine population, suggesting that they represent restricted events of interspecies transmission.

Interestingly, 90.3% of equine RVA strains typed around the world carry a P [12] P-genotype [62], suggesting that the receptor used by RVA in the epithelial cells of the equine intestine might be quite unique and an specific variant of VP4 is needed to successfully infect horses and persist in the species. Pathogenesis studies in infected foals are needed to elucidate this interesting unique feature.

The combination G3P [12] in the prevalent strain and widely distributed in Thoroughbred horses, being detected in 12 countries within all continents, except Africa [62] (Figure 8). The combinationG14P [12] became predominant in the nineties initially in Japan and was then detected in other countries like Argentina, Ireland and the UK [62].

The G14 genotype is restricted to equine RVA and according tophylogenetic analysis based on nucleotide sequences it appears to constitute a cluster within the G3 genotype, with percentages of identity higher than 80%, the cut off value for a new genotype, according to the RCWG(Matthijnssens et al., 2008a,b).However, when the phylogenetic analysis was performed with the deduced aa sequences, the G14 equine RVA strains clearly clustered as an independent G type.

In fact, the alignment of the aa sequences showed that the genotype G3 of the Argentinean Equine RVA strains is well represented by the VP7 protein ofH2 (G3 subtype A), the strain included in the vaccine, while the G14 strains showed nine mutations within the antigenic regions, including the generation of new glycosylation sites, compared with that of the H2 strain. This observation is in concordance with cross-neutralization assay results previously published [70] that established G14 as a different serotype from G3, but serologically more related than the other serotypes.

After the creation of the RCWG, the genome constellation of the RVA strains detected in horses from several European, American and African countries was studied [62, 71], the configuration of the backbone genes of equine RVA strains show a peculiar conserved composition:G3/G14-P [12]-I2/I6-R2-C2-M3-A10-N2-T3-E2/E12-H7 (Table 3).

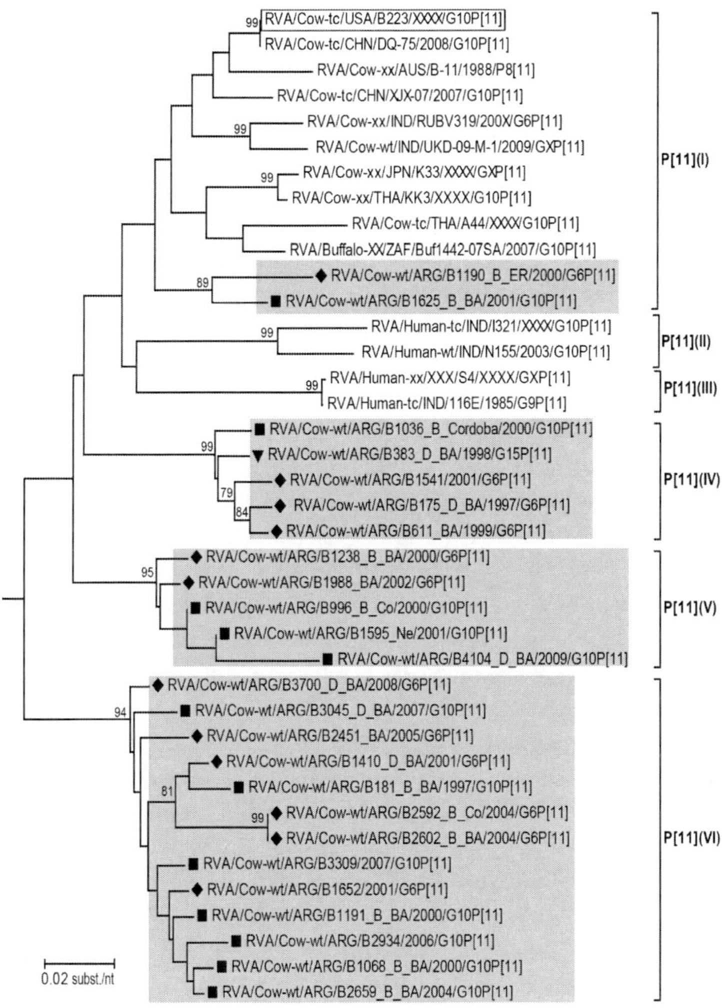

Figure 8. Bioinformatic analyses of the P [11] genotype. (A) The phylogenetic tree was constructed using the Poisson model and Neighbor-Joining methods using the program MEGA5. Bootstrap values are shown at the branch nodes. The lineages are indicated at the right hand side. The Argentinean strains isolated are shown in grey boxes and the vaccines strains are indicated with open squares. In the Argentinean strains: name of the strain, type of exploitation and province of collection are shown. Abbreviations: D/B, Dairy or Beef; BA, Buenos Aires; Co, Cordoba; ER, Entre Rios; Ne, Neuquén; ♦, G6P [11]; ■ G10P [11]; ▼G15P [11].

Remarkable geographic patterns can be highlighted like the E12 NSP4 genotype exclusively carried by the Argentinean equine RVA strains, shared with other RVA found in camelids, bovine and goats from Argentina [1, 15, 71, 72]. The H-1 constellation suggests its porcine origin (G5-P [7]-I5-R1-C1-M1-A8-N1-T1-E1-H1) [73], while E3198 strains share the genetic composition of feline/canine (G3-P [3]-I3-R3-C3-M3-A9-N3-T3-E3-H6) RVA strains, respectively [69].

Several equine RVA inactivated vaccines for the prevention of rotavirus diarrhea in foals have been developed. Pregnant mares are vaccinated in the last third of pregnancy to provide passive transfer of antibodies to foals against equine RVA. Argentina was the first country with a licensed vaccine to prevent equine RVA diarrhea in foals in the local market. The vaccine was formulated with the prototype H2 (G3P [12]), simian rotavirus SA11 (G3 P [2]), and bovine rotavirus NCDV-Lincoln (G6 P [1]) strains, in aqueous adjuvant (Alumina gel) [74]. Later on, A vaccine developed in the USA using the strain H2 (P [12]G3a) (Fort Dodge Animal Health, USA) was initially licensed in the USA, Great Britain and Ireland and is now commercially available in several countries [75].The systematic application of the Argentinean vaccine to the pregnant mares, since 1996, has drastically reduced the incidence of equine RVA diarrhea in foals in the most important polo and thoroughbred horse farms in the country.

The outbreaks for equine RVA decreased, and no virus was detected in farms that submitted samples of diarrheic foals to the service during the years 2001 and 2002. However, in the years 2006 and 2007, an increase in diarrhea cases positive for equine RVA coincided with a change in the prevalent genotype, from G3 to G14, which was not included in the vaccine [2]. Similar results of temporal changes in the circulating genotypes, after introduction of G3P [12] inactivated vaccine were observed in Japan (Tsunemitsu et al., 2001) and in Ireland (Collins et al., 2008). These results suggest that the equine RV vaccine should be updated according to the increase in the circulation of G14 strains. However, a recent study conducted with other vaccines, formulated with the strain HO-5 (P [12] G3b), licensed in Japan since 2000, demonstrated that this vaccine induced high neutralizing antibody titers to the homologous virus G3b and also a lower titer of neutralizing antibodies to the heterologous strain G14 [76]. Finally, the conservation of the P type of the equine RVA, suggests that the development of a recombinant subunit vaccine based on VP8* P [12] would be an excellent prevention strategy to avoid breaking the immune barrier originated for the cyclic switch in the G types, when using inactivated vaccines.

Table 3. Gene constellation of Equine RVA strains

Strain Name	VP7	VP4	VP6	VP1	VP2	VP3	NSP1	NSP2	NSP3	NSP4	NSP5
RVA/Horse-wt/ARG/E30/1993	G3	P [12]	I6	R2	C2	M3	A10	N2	T3	E12	H7
RVA/Horse-wt/ARG/E403/2006/G14P [12] RVA/Horse-wt/A RG/E4040/2008/G14P [12]	G14	P [12]	I2	R2	C2	M3	A10	N2	T3	E12	H7
RVA/Horse-wt/ARG/E3198/2008/G3P [3]	G3	P [3]	I3	R3	C3	M3	A9	N3	T3	E3	H6
RVA/Horse-wt/IRL/03V4954 /2003/G3P [12]	G3	P [12]	I6	R2	C2	M3	A10	N2	T3	E2	H7
RVA/Horse-wt/I RL/04V2024 /2004/G14P [12], RVA /Horse-wt/ZA F/EqRV-SA1/2006/G14P [12]	G14	P [12]	I2	R2	C2	M3	A10	N2	T3	E2	H7
RVA/Horse-tc/ GBR/H-1/1975/G5P9 [7]	G5	P [7]	I5	R1	C1	M1	A8	N1	T1	E1	H1
RVA/Horse-tc/ GBR/L33 8/1991 G13P [18]	G13	P [18]	I6	R9	C9	M6	A6	N9	T12	E14	H11

Extracted from Mathijnssenss, 2011;Miño, 2013 and Baley, 2013.

Rotavirus in Camelids

Members of the Camelidae family are classified as Old world camelids and new world or South American camelids. The Bactrian camel and Dromedary are Old world camelids, while the wild species vicuña (*Vicugnavicugna*) and guanaco(*Lama guanicoe*), and their derived domestic counterparts alpaca (*Vicugnapacos*) and llama (*Lamaglama*) are the four species of native camelids from South America.

All species of camelids are susceptible to RVA infection, since all surveyed populations are seropositive for antibodies to the virus [77-79]. RVA has been detected in feces of domestic alpacas and llamas with diarrhea in Peru, Chile and USA (Berrios, 1988; Lopez et al., 2011) [5].

The first RVA typed in wild SACs was reported by our group of research in two guanacos crias with severe diarrhea sampled in 1998 and 1999 in the Argentinean Patagonia Region [80].

The strains were typed as G8P [1] and G8 [14] [81]. In 2012, we reported the detection of RVA in a healthy cria of wild vicugna from the Andean Puna, this strain was typed as G8P [14] [4]. In 2011 we were able to detect RVA in 57 out of 1423 samples from alpacas crias from Puno, Peru(Badaracco and Cordero, unpublished data). Three representative strains were typed as G8P [1], G8P [14] and G3P [14]. The complete genome of all the RVA detected in SACs from Argentina and Peru were obtained in collaboration with Jelle Mathijnssens, Van Ranstand the RCWG, at the Rega Institute, Belgium (Table 4).

Regarding old world camelids, Papp et. al. (2012) conducted an epidemiologic survey between October 2008 and December 2010 in five farms of Arabian camels (*Camelusdromedarius*) in Kuwait, and found8 RVA positives among 517 stool samples.

Of these eight positives, five samples were from diarrheic animals of 4 months of age, and three samples were from asymptomatic animals of 3 years of age. One strain, RVA/Camel-wt/KUW/s21/2010/G10P [15], collected from a 4month old dromedary calf with diarrhea was subsequently available for complete genome analysis (Table 4).

The genome constellation of the SACs (guanacos, vicugnas and two strains from alpacas) showed a similar structure G8-P [1]/P [14]-I2-R2/R5-C2-M2-N2-T6-E3/12-H3 [4], suggesting that this constellation in specific SACs are genetically related tithe variants found in bovines, buffaloes, antelopes, goat and sheep, all belonging to the order of *Artiodactyla* [15, 72].

Table 4. Gene constellation of RVA detected in member of the *Camelidae* Family

Strain	VP7	VP4	VP6	VP1	VP2	VP3	NSP1	NSP2	NSP3	NSP4	NSP5
RVA/alpaca-wt/PER/356/2010/G3P [14]	G3	P [14]	I2	R5	C3	M3	A17	N3	T6	E3	H3
RVA/alpaca-wt/PER/1115/2010/G8P [1]	G8	P [1]	I2	R2	C2	M2	A17	N2	T6	E3	H3
RVA/alpaca-wt/PER/562/2010/G8P [14]	G8	P [14]	I2	R5	C2	M2	A17	N2	T6	E3	H3
RVA/vicugna-wt/ARG/75/2010/G8P [14]	G8	P [14]	I2	R2	C2	M2		N2	T6	E3	
RVA/Guanaco-wt/ARG/Chubut/1999/G8P [14]	G8	P [14]	I2	R5	C2	M2	A11	N2	T6	E12	H3
RVA/Guanaco-wt/ARG/RioNegro/1998/G8P [1]	G8	P [1]	I2	R5	C2	M2	A13	N2	T6	E12	H3
RVA/Camel-wt/KUW/s21/2010/G10P [15]	G10	P [15]		R1	C2			N2	T2	E15	H3
RVA/Antelope-wt/ZAF/RC-18/2008/G6P [14]	G6	P [14]	I2	R2	C2	M2	A11	N2	T6	E2	H3

Interestingly the genotype of the NSP4 protein varies from the guanacos living in Patagonia that was classified as E12 as the other RVA found in bovine and goats in the Pampean region, both at sea level, while the RVA detected in the vicugna and the alpacas from the Andean Puna from Argentina or Peru (around 2,000 meter over sea level) were typed as E3, thus NSP4 is acting as a geographical marker (in terms of area apart in distance and in altitude). Additionally, the partial sequence data of the RVA strain G10P [15] detected in a dromedary (Camelusdromedarius, family Camelidae) from Kuwait revealed quite different constellation with a new NSP4 genotype E15 [8]. Finally, the third sequence from alpaca G3P [14] represents an interspecies transmission probably from a feline/canine or human origin (Table 4).

The analysis of old word and new world camelids provided interesting data to RVA epidemiology, diversity and evolution. Further surveys of all the species of this family living in their native environments are encouraged to improve our knowledge regarding RVA infection in camelids.

Rotavirus in Goats and Sheep

Goat production is an important economic activity of small farmers, mainly in poor rural areas in Argentina where the goat population is approximately 4,257,000animals. Goat husbandry systems can have different production purposes including meat, fiber, skin for leather, milk and cheese. Ovine production is important in Argentina, accounting for more than 15,000,000 heads, mainly concentrated in the Patagonia region [27].

Worldwide information regarding caprine and ovine RVA is scarce but there are several reports from the nineties which indicate that goats are susceptible to infection with group A, B and C rotaviruses [7, 82-85] while RVA and RVB had been detected in lambs [6, 86-90].

Kaminjolo, et al. (1994) found RVA in goat kids samples in Trinidad [85]. Da Costa Mendes reported the first detection of RVA in goats from South Africa, in 1994 [7, 84]. Two years later, Muñoz, et al. (1996) reported the detection of RVA and RVB in diarrheic goat kids and RVC innon-diarrheic goat kids from a survey conducted of goat kids aged 1-45 days, from Spain [83, 86].Rotavirus group B was also reported in goats from France [82]. Lee et al. first reported caprine RVA with aG3P5 [3] genotype in Korea [91]. In 2011 Alkan et al. characterized a G8P [1] I2E2 strain causing severe diarrhea in goats from Turkey [3].

Table 5. Gene constellation of RVA detected in goats and lambs

Strain	VP7	VP4	VP6	VP1	VP2	VP3	NSP1	NSP2	NSP3	NSP4	NSP5
RVA/goat-wt/ARG/Cabra/2011/G8P [1]	G8	P [1]	I2	R5	C2	M2	A3	N2	T6	E12	H3
RVA/Sheep-tc/ESP/OVR762/2002/G8P [14]	G8	P [14]	I2	R2	C2	M2	A11	N2	T6	E2	H3
RVA/Sheep-tc/CHN/Lamb-NT/XXXX/G10P [15]	G10	P [15]	I10	R2	C2	M2	A11	N2	T6	E2	H3
RVA/Sheep-xx/CHN/CC0812-1/2008/G10P [15]	G10	P [15]	I10	R2	C2	M2	A11	N2	T6	E2	H3
RVA/Goat-tc/BGD/GO34/1999/G6P [1]	G6	P [1]	I2	R2	C2	M2	A11	N2	T6	E2	H3
RVA/Goat-tc/TUR/Kirklareli/2007/G8 [1]	G8	P [1]	I2							E2	
GRV/Cap	G3	P [3]								E3	
Cap455/Cap	G6	P [14]									

There are only two complete genome constellations of caprine RVA, one from India [54] and the one reported by our group in Argentina [72] Table 5.

Regarding RVA circulation in lambs, three complete genome constellations are available, two strains from China and one from Spain [6, 87, 89] Table 5.

The complete genome sequence of the caprine and ovine RVA rotavirus (GAR) showed the following G6/G8/G10-P [1]/ [14]-I2/10-R2/5-C2-M2-A3/11-N2-T6-E12/2-H3 genotypes, respectively.

These gene constellations point to a common evolutionary origin of caprine and ovine RVA with bovine, antelope, guanaco and camels. It is interesting to note that camel RVA from Kuwait and sheep from China shared the same G/P combination G10P [15] (Table 4 and 5). Conversely, the Argentinean caprine strain 0040 is more closely related to the RVA detected in guanacos than the RVA detected in other goats and possesses the R5 and E12 genotypes found only in animals from Argentina and alpacas from Peru [2, 15, 72].

Overall, the data summarized that rotavirus broadly circulated in the populations of goat and ovines cause diarrhea, however the impact of the infection in the production need further studies. Further analyses of caprineand ovine RVA strains around the world are still needed to properly understand their genetic diversity.

Final Considerations

Rotavirus is a ubiquitous pathogen affecting a large variety of animal species.

The continuous survey and molecular characterization of the strains circulating in wild and domestic animals around the world have generated interesting data for a better understanding of the genetic diversity and mechanisms of evolution of viruses with segmented genomes.

References

[1] Garaicoechea, L., et al., Molecular characterization of bovine rotavirus circulating in beef and dairy herds in Argentina during a 10-year period (1994-2003). *Vet. Microbiol.,* 2006. 118(1-2): p. 1-11.

[2] Garaicoechea, L., et al., Molecular characterization of equine rotaviruses circulating in Argentinean foals during a 17-year surveillance period (1992-2008). *Vet. Microbiol*., 2011. 148(2-4): p. 150-60.

[3] Alkan, F., et al., A large outbreak of enteritis in goat flocks in Marmara, Turkey, by G8P [1] group A rotaviruses. *Arch. Virol.,* 2012.

[4] Badaracco, A., et al., Discovery and molecular characterization of a group A rotavirus strain detected in an Argentinean vicuna (Vicugnavicugna). *Vet. Microbiol*., 2012. 161(3-4): p. 247-54.

[5] Cebra, C.K., et al., Potential pathogens in feces from unweaned llamas and alpacas with diarrhea. *J. Am. Vet. Med. Assoc*., 2003. 223(12): p. 1806-8.

[6] Ciarlet, M., et al., Genomic characterization of a novel group A lamb rotavirus isolated in Zaragoza, Spain. *Virus Genes*, 2008. 37(2): p. 250-65.

[7] da Costa Mendes, V.M., et al., Rotavirus in Saanen goats. *J. S. Afr. Vet. Assoc*., 1994. 65(3): p. 132-3.

[8] Papp, H., et al., Novel NSP4 genotype in a camel G10P [15] rotavirus strain. *Acta. Microbiol. Immunol. Hung.,* 2012. 59(3): p. 411-21.

[9] Estes, M.K. and A.Z. Kapikian, Rotaviruses, in Field's Virology D.M. Knipe and P.M. Howley, Editors. 2007, Lippincott Williams & Wilkins: Philadelphia. p. 1917-1974.

[10] Matthijnssens, J., et al., VP6-sequence-based cutoff values as a criterion for rotavirus species demarcation. *Arch. Virol*., 2012. 157(6): p. 1177-82.

[11] Saif, L.J. and F.M. Fernandez, Group A rotavirus veterinary vaccines. *J. Infect. Dis*., 1996. 174 Suppl. 1: p. S98-106.

[12] Matthijnssens, J., et al., Uniformity of rotavirus strain nomenclature proposed by the Rotavirus Classification Working Group (RCWG). *Arch. Virol*., 2011. 156(8): p. 1397-413.

[13] Matthijnssens, J., et al., Recommendations for the classification of group A rotaviruses using all 11 genomic RNA segments. *Arch. Virol.,* 2008. 153(8): p. 1621-9.

[14] Matthijnssens, J., et al., Group A rotavirus universal mass vaccination: how and to what extent will selective pressure influence the prevalence of rotavirus genotypes? *Expert Rev. Vaccines*, 2012. 11(11): p. 1347-54.

[15] Matthijnssens, J., et al., Are human P [14] rotavirus strains the result of interspecies transmissions from sheep or other ungulates that belong to the mammalian order Artiodactyla? *J. Virol.*, 2009. 83(7): p. 2917-29.

[16] Bendali, F., et al., Risk factors associated with diarrhea in newborn calves. *Vet. Res.*, 1999. 30(5): p. 509-22.

[17] Makoschey, B., et al., Neonatal health in calves--comprehensive solutions for complex enteric disorders. Berl Munch Tierarztl Wochenschr, 2009. 122(9-10): p. 398-408.

[18] Blanchard, P.C., Diagnostics of dairy and beef cattle diarrhea. *Vet. Clin. North Am. Food Anim. Pract.,* 2012. 28(3): p. 443-64.

[19] Chang, K.O., et al., Detection of group B rotaviruses in fecal samples from diarrheic calves and adult cows and characterization of their VP7 genes. *J. Clin. Microbiol.*, 1997. 35(8): p. 2107-10.

[20] Ghosh, S., et al., Molecular characterization of the VP1, VP2, VP4, VP6, NSP1 and NSP2 genes of bovine group B rotaviruses: identification of a novel VP4 genotype. *Arch. Virol.*, 2010. 155(2): p. 159-67.

[21] Tsunemitsu, H., et al., Molecular characterization of the major capsid protein VP6 of bovine group B rotavirus and its use in seroepidemiology. *J. Gen. Virol.*, 2005. 86(Pt 9): p. 2569-75.

[22] Tsunemitsu, H., et al., First detection of bovine group B rotavirus in Japan and sequence of its VP7 gene. *Arch. Virol.,* 1999. 144(4): p. 805-15.

[23] Park, S.I., et al., Genetically diverse group C rotaviruses cause sporadic infection in Korean calves. *J. Vet. Med. Sci.*, 2011. 73(4): p. 479-82.

[24] Cho, Y.I., et al., Case-control study of microbiological etiology associated with calf diarrhea. *Vet. Microbiol.,* 2013. 166(3-4): p. 375-85.

[25] Park, S.J., et al., Detection and molecular characterization of calf diarrhea bovine coronaviruses circulating in South Korea during 2004-2005. *Zoonoses Public Health*, 2007. 54(6-7): p. 223-30.

[26] Bartels, C.J., et al., Prevalence, prediction and risk factors of enteropathogens in normal and non-normal feces of young Dutch dairy calves. *Prev. Vet. Med.*, 2010. 93(2-3): p. 162-9.

[27] INDEC, Encuesta Nacional Agropecuaria (ENA 2001). 2002, Intituto Nacional de Estadísticas y Censos (INDEC). Secretaria de Política Económica - Ministerio de Economía: Buenos Aires.

[28] Badaracco, A., et al., Bovine rotavirus strains circulating in beef and dairy herds in Argentina from 2004 to 2010. *Vet. Microbiol.,* 2011. 158(3-4): p. 394-9.

[29] Alfieri, A.A., et al., Frequency of group A rotavirus in diarrheic calves in Brazilian cattle herds, 1998-2002. *Trop. Anim. Health Prod.*, 2006. 38(7-8): p. 521-6.

[30] Papp, H., et al., Review of group A rotavirus strains reported in swine and cattle. *Vet. Microbiol.,* 2013. 165(3-4): p. 190-9.

[31] Matthijnssens, J., et al., Full genome-based classification of rotaviruses reveals a common origin between human Wa-Like and porcine rotavirus strains and human DS-1-like and bovine rotavirus strains. *J.Virol.*, 2008. 82(7): p. 3204-19.

[32] Kindler, E., et al., Analysis of rotavirus species diversity and evolution including the newly determined full-length genome sequences of rotavirus F and G. *Infect. Genet.Evol.*, 2013. 14: p. 58-67.

[33] Trojnar, E., et al., Identification of an avian group A rotavirus containing a novel VP4 gene with a close relationship to those of mammalian rotaviruses. *J. Gen.Virol.*, 2013. 94(Pt 1): p. 136-42.

[34] Abe, M., et al., Whole genome characterization of new bovine rotavirus G21P [29] and G24P [33] strains provide evidence for interspecies transmission. *J. Gen.Virol.,* 2011. 92(Pt 4): p. 952-60.

[35] Alfieri, A.F., et al., G and P genotypes of group A rotavirus strains circulating in calves in Brazil, 1996-1999. *Vet. Microbiol.,* 2004. 99(3-4): p. 167-73.

[36] Alkan, F., et al., Distribution of G (VP7) and P (VP4) genotypes of group A bovine rotaviruses from Turkish calves with diarrhea, 1997-2008. *Vet. Microbiol.,* 2010. 141(3-4): p. 231-7.

[37] Cashman, O., et al., Changing profile of the bovine rotavirus G6 population in the south of Ireland from 2002 to 2009. *Vet. Microbiol.,* 2010. 146(3-4): p. 238-44.

[38] Kapikian, A.a.C., Rotaviruses (Cap 55), in Virology, D.M.K. B. N. Fields, P. M. Howley, Editor. 1996, Lippincott-Raven: Philadelphia.

[39] Monini, M., et al., Molecular characterization of bovine rotavirus strains circulating in northern Italy, 2003-2005. *Vet. Microbiol.,* 2008. 129(3-4): p. 384-9.

[40] Badaracco, A., et al., Phylogenetic analyses of typical bovine rotavirus genotypes G6, G10, P [5] and P [11] circulating in Argentinean beef and dairy herds. *Infect. Genet.Evol.*, 2013. 18: p. 18-30.

[41] Banyai, K., et al., Genetic variability among serotype G6 human rotaviruses: identification of a novel lineage isolated in Hungary. *J. Med. Virol.,* 2003. 71(1): p. 124-34.

[42] Martella, V., et al., Molecular analysis of the VP7, VP4, VP6, NSP4, and NSP5/6 genes of a buffalo rotavirus strain: identification of the rare P [3] rhesus rotavirus-like VP4 gene allele. *J.Clin.Microbiol.*, 2003. 41(12): p. 5665-75.

[43] Parra, G.I., et al., Phylogenetic analysis of porcine rotavirus in Argentina: increasing diversity of G4 strains and evidence of interspecies transmission. *Vet. Microbiol.,* 2008. 126(1-3): p. 243-50.

[44] Matsuda, Y., et al., Two-way cross-neutralization mediated by a shared P (VP4) serotype between bovine rotavirus strains with distinct G (VP7) serotypes. *J. Clin. Microbiol.*, 1993. 31(2): p. 354-8.

[45] Chang, K.O., A.V. Parwani, and L.J. Saif, Comparative sequence analysis of the VP7 genes of G6, G8 and G10 bovine group A rotaviruses and further characterization of G6 subtypes. *Arch. Virol.,* 2000. 145(4): p. 725-37.

[46] Volotao, E.M., et al., Rotavirus surveillance in the city of Rio de Janeiro-Brazil during 2000-2004: detection of unusual strains with G8P [4] or G10P [9] specificities. *J. Med. Virol.,* 2006. 78(2): p. 263-72.

[47] Manuja, B.K., et al., A novel genomic constellation (G10P [3]) of group A rotavirus detected from buffalo calves in northern India. *Virus Res.,* 2008. 138(1-2): p. 36-42.

[48] Bhandari, N., et al., Safety and immunogenicity of two live attenuated human rotavirus vaccine candidates, 116E and I321, in infants: results of a randomised controlled trial. *Vaccine*, 2006. 24(31-32): p. 5817-23.

[49] Esona, M.D., et al., Genomic characterization of human rotavirus G10 strains from the African Rotavirus Network: relationship to animal rotaviruses. *Infect. Genet. Evol.*, 2011. 11(1): p. 237-41.

[50] Ramani, S., et al., Whole genome characterization of reassortantG10P [11] strain (N155) from a neonate with symptomatic rotavirus infection: identification of genes of human and animal rotavirus origin. *J. Clin. Virol.*, 2009. 45(3): p. 237-44.

[51] Ramos Caruzo, T.A., et al., Molecular characterization of G and P-types bovine rotavirus strains from Goiás, Brazil: high frequency of mixed P-type infections. *Mem. Inst. Oswaldo Cruz, Rio de Janeiro.*, 2010. 105(8): p. 1040-1043.

[52] Nakagomi, O., et al., Naturally occurring dual infection with human and bovine rotaviruses as suggested by the recovery of G1P8 and G1P5 rotaviruses from a single patient. *Arch. Virol.,* 1994. 137(3-4): p. 381-8.

[53] Park, S.I., et al., Reassortment among bovine, porcine and human rotavirus strains results in G8P [7] and G6P [7] strains isolated from cattle in South Korea. *Vet. Microbiol.,* 2011. 152(1-2): p. 55-66.

[54] Ghosh, S., et al., Complete genome constellation of a caprine group A rotavirus strain reveals common evolution with ruminant and human rotavirus strains. *J. Gen.Virol.*, 2010. 91(Pt 9): p. 2367-73.

[55] Matthijnssens, J., et al., Molecular and biological characterization of the 5 human-bovine rotavirus (WC3)-based reassortant strains of the pentavalent rotavirus vaccine, RotaTeq. *Virology*, 2010. 403(2): p. 111-27.

[56] O'Shea, H., et al., Complete genomic sequence analyses of the first group A giraffe rotavirus reveals close evolutionary relationship with rotaviruses infecting other members of the Artiodactyla. *Vet. Microbiol.,* 2014. 170(1-2): p. 151-6.

[57] Doan, Y.H., et al., Identification by full-genome analysis of a bovine rotavirus transmitted directly to and causing diarrhea in a human child. *J. Clin. Microbiol.*, 2013. 51(1): p. 182-9.

[58] Matthijnssens, J., et al., Multiple reassortment and interspecies transmission events contribute to the diversity of feline, canine and feline/canine-like human group A rotavirus strains. *Infect. Genet.Evol.,* 2011. 11(6): p. 1396-406.

[59] Jere, K.C., et al., Whole genome sequence analyses of three African bovine rotaviruses reveal that they emerged through multiple reassortment events between rotaviruses from different mammalian species. *Vet. Microbiol.,* 2012. 159(1-2): p. 245-50.

[60] Flewett, T.H., Electron microscopy in the diagnosis of infectious diarrhea. *J. Am. Vet. Med. Assoc.*, 1978. 173(5 Pt 2): p. 538-43.

[61] Bailey, K.E., J.R. Gilkerson, and G.F. Browning, Equine rotaviruses--current understanding and continuing challenges. *Vet. Microbiol.,* 2013. 167(1-2): p. 135-44.

[62] Papp, H., et al., Global distribution of group A rotavirus strains in horses: a systematic review. *Vaccine,* 2013. 31(48): p. 5627-33.

[63] Kapikian, A.Z., Overview of viral gastroenteritis. *Arch.Virol. Suppl.,* 1996. 12: p. 7-19.

[64] Dwyer, R.M., Rotaviral diarrhea. *Vet. Clin. North Am. Equine Pract.,* 1993. 9(2): p. 311-9.

[65] Browning, G.F., et al., Serological and genomic characterization of L338, a novel equine group A rotavirus G serotype. *J. Gen.Virol.*, 1991. 72 (Pt 5): p. 1059-64.
[66] Hoshino, Y., et al., Isolation and characterization of an equine rotavirus. *J.Clin.Microbiol.*, 1983. 18(3): p. 585-91.
[67] Isa, P., et al., Survey of equine rotaviruses shows conservation of one P genotype in background of two G genotypes. *Arch. Virol.,* 1996. 141(9): p. 1601-12.
[68] Imagawa, H., et al., Genetic analysis of equine rotavirus by RNA-RNA hybridization. *J.Clin.Microbiol.*, 1994. 32(8): p. 2009-12.
[69] Mino, S., et al., Equine G3P [3] rotavirus strain E3198 related to simian RRV and feline/canine-like rotaviruses based on complete genome analyses. *Vet. Microbiol.,* 2013. 161(3-4): p. 239-46.
[70] Ciarlet, M., et al. Equine rotaviruses with G14 serotype specificity circulate among Venezuelan horses. *J.Clin.Microbiol.,* 1994. 32(10): p. 2609-12.
[71] Matthijnssens, J., et al., Complete molecular genome analyses of equine rotavirus A strains from different continents reveal several novel genotypes and a largely conserved genotype constellation. *J. Gen.Virol.,* 2012. 93(Pt 4): p. 866-75.
[72] LougeUriarte, E.L., et al., The first caprine rotavirus detected in Argentina displays genomic features resembling virus strains infecting members of the Bovidae and Camelidae. *Vet. Microbiol.,* 2014. 171(1-2): p. 189-97.
[73] Ghosh, S., T. Shintani, and N. Kobayashi, Evidence for the porcine origin of equine rotavirus strain H-1. *Vet. Microbiol.,* 2012. 158(3-4): p. 410-4.
[74] Barrandeguy, M., et al., Prevention of rotavirus diarrhea in foals by parenteral vaccination of the mares: field trial. *Dev. Biol. Stand.*, 1998. 92: p. 253-7.
[75] Powell, D.G., et al., Field study of the safety, immunogenicity, and efficacy of an inactivated equine rotavirus vaccine. *J. Am. Vet. Med. Assoc.,* 1997. 211(2): p. 193-8.
[76] Nemoto, M., et al., Antibody response in vaccinated pregnant mares to recent G3BP [12] and G14P [12] equine rotaviruses. *Acta. Vet. Scand.,* 2012. 54: p. 63.
[77] Marcoppido, G., et al., Study of the kinetics of antibodies titres against viral pathogens and detection of rotavirus and parainfluenza 3 infections

in captive crias of guanacos (Lama guanicoe). *TransboundEmerg. Dis.*, 2011. 58(1): p. 37-43.

[78] Marcoppido, G., V. Parreno, and B. Vila, Antibodies to pathogenic livestock viruses in a wild vicuna (Vicugnavicugna) population in the Argentinean Andean altiplano. *J. Wildl. Dis.*, 2010. 46(2): p. 608-14.

[79] Puntel, M., [Seroprevalence of viral infections in llamas (Lama glama) in the Republic of Argentina]. *Rev. Argent. Microbiol.*, 1997. 29(1): p. 38-46.

[80] Parreno, V., et al., First isolation of rotavirus associated with neonatal diarrhea in guanacos (Lama guanicoe) in the Argentinean Patagonia region. *J. Vet. Med. B. Infect. Dis. Vet. Public Health*, 2001. 48(9): p. 713-20.

[81] Parreno, V., et al., Molecular characterization of the first isolation of rotavirus in guanacos (Lama guanicoe). *Arch. Virol.*, 2004. 149(12): p. 2465-71.

[82] Gueguen, C., et al., Caprine and bovine B rotaviruses in western France: group identification by Northern hybridization. *Vet. Res.*, 1996. 27(2): p. 171-6.

[83] Munoz, M., et al., An outbreak of diarrhea associated with atypical rotaviruses in goat kids. *Res. Vet. Sci.*, 1995. 59(2): p. 180-2.

[84] Mendes, V.M., et al., Isolation and preliminary characterization of a caprine rotavirus. *Onderstepoort J. Vet. Res.*, 1994. 61(4): p. 291-4.

[85] Kaminjolo, J.S. and A.A. Adesiyun, Rotavirus infection in calves, piglets, lambs and goat kids in Trinidad. *Br. Vet. J.*, 1994. 150(3): p. 293-9.

[86] Munoz, M., et al., Role of enteric pathogens in the aetiology of neonatal diarrhea in lambs and goat kids in Spain. *Epidemiol. Infect.*, 1996. 117(1): p. 203-11.

[87] Shen, S., B. Burke, and U. Desselberger, Nucleotide sequences of the VP4 and VP7 genes of a Chinese lamb rotavirus: evidence for a new P type in a G10 type virus. *Virology*, 1993. 197(1): p. 497-500.

[88] Wani, S.A., et al., Evidence of rotavirus associated with neonatal lamb diarrhea in India. *Trop. Anim. Health Prod.*, 2004. 36(1): p. 27-32.

[89] Chen, Y., et al., Whole genome sequencing of lamb rotavirus and comparative analysis with other mammalian rotaviruses. *Virus Genes*, 2009. 38(2): p. 302-10.

[90] Galindo-Cardiel, I., et al., Novel group A rotavirus G8 P [1] as primary cause of an ovine diarrheic syndrome outbreak in weaned lambs. *Vet. Microbiol.,* 2011. 149(3-4): p. 467-71.

[91] Lee, J.B., et al., Isolation, serologic and molecular characterization of the first G3 caprine rotavirus. *Arch. Virol.*, 2003. 148(4): p. 643-57.

Remarkably, heavy chain antibodies also occur in shark, wobbegong, and spotted ratfish and are named Ig-NAR. These ancestral antibodies have a variable domain, known as VNAR, for antigen binding. Although the sequences of the variable domains of Ig-NARs (VNAR) and camel HCAbs (V_HH) are quite diverse, they show a surprising structural and functional convergent evolution (Figure 2) [3].

V_HH fragments can be expressed as recombinant proteins and represent the smallest molecule present in nature capable of antigen recognition and biding. Due to their small size, recombinant V_HH molecules have been shown to act as strong enzyme inhibitors, reaching enzyme pockets and hidden targets not accessible to conventional antibodies. Other interesting properties are the resistance to extreme pH and high temperatures, better tissue penetration and the potential to cross the blood-brain barrier. These properties allow the development of a new generation of monoclonal recombinant antibody therapies for cancer, autoimmune disease, diagnosis and treatment of infectious diseases, and many other biotechnological applications [2, 4].

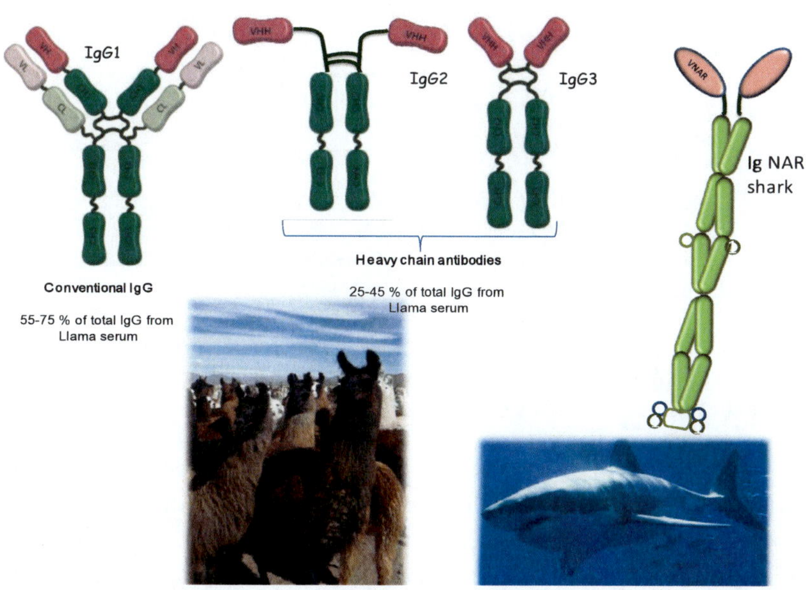

Figure 1. Schematic representation of antibodies present in sera of camelids: Conventional antibodies (IgG1) containing two light chains and two heavy chains and two types of homodimeric heavy chain antibodies (HCAbs), IgG2 and IgG3, which comprises only heavy chains; each H chain contains a VH, hinge and two constant domains. Homodimeric shark antibody devoid of light chain (Ig-NAR).

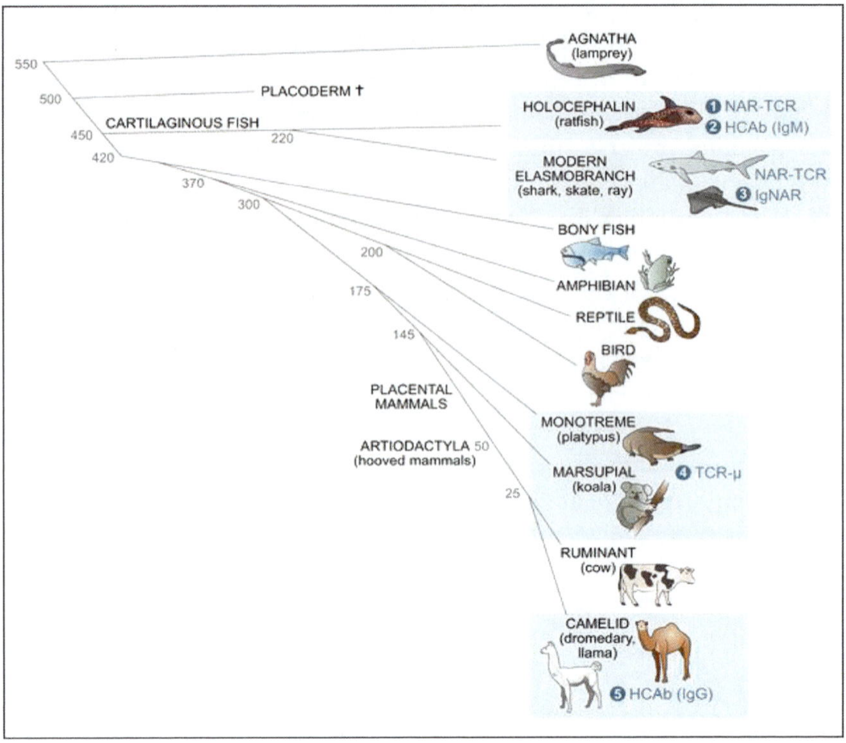

Flajnik MF, Deschacht N, Muyldermans S (2011) A Case Of Convergence: Why Did a Simple Alternative to Canonical Antibodies Arise in Sharks and Camels? PLoS Biol 9(8): e1001120. doi:10.1371/journal.pbio.1001120 http://www.plosbiology.org/article/info:doi/10.1371/journal.pbio.1001120.

Figure 2. Simplified vertebrate phylogenetic tree showing those taxa possessing single domain Immunoglobulines or TCRs. Blue boxes display animal groups shown or predicted to have single-domain variable regions.

As an example of its surprising behavior, V_HH directed to Group A Rotavirus (RVA) inner capsid VP6 protein was capable of neutralizing the virus infection *in vitro*, independently of the viral serotype, and of protecting mice [5–7] and gnotobiotic piglets [8] from the threat of human RVA. Anti-RVA V_HH are especially convenient for oral therapies, given their low immunogenicity when administered as a milk supplement [8]. Furthermore, anti VP6 V_HH antibodies were shown to decrease the stool output of RVA induced diarrhea in human male infants in a clinical trial carried out in Bangladesh [9]. V_HH antibodies against other viral diseases have been developed (foot and mouth disease, influenza, rabies, respiratory syncytial virus, porcine retrovirus, HIV) and the publications were reviewed by Vanlandschoot, Stortelers et al., representing a promising next-generation biological platform for passive immunity [10].

Heavy Chain Antibody Isotypes and Structural Features

The absence of L chains and the lack of the CH1 domain in the H chain are key characteristics of camelid HCAbs. The more compact architecture and smaller size of HCAbs - with a molecular weight of 90,000 compared to 150,000 Da for conventional antibodies - give a better adapted structure to access hidden epitopes. The percentage of HCAbs and conventional IgG in the sera of camelids is variable. In camels, it might reach 50–80%, while in South American Camelid species, the total concentration of HCAbs reaches up to 10–25%. The shorter distance between the two paratopes within one HCAb due to the absence of CH1 domain might reduce their ability to cross-link antigens. There are two isotypes of HCAbs, IgG3 with a short hinge and IgG2 with a long hinge region that might form an extended spacer that structurally replaces the CH1 region (Figure 1). Both types of antibodies can be separated by sequential affinity chromatography using protein G and protein A [2].

Structure of a V_HH (Variable Domain of Heavy Chain Antibodies)

The V_HH domain is composed of three hypervariable regions that fold, forming a continuous surface, complementary to the surface of the antigen epitope. These regions are named complementarity-determining regions (CDR1, CDR2 and CDR3). Each of these variable regions is surrounded by more conserved framework regions (FR1 to FR4) (Figure 3).

Direct inspection of the alignment of V_HH amino acid sequences indicates that the structural organization of the FR and CDR regions is similar to the VH of the conventional antibodies. However, many important differences were observed. All V_HH domains possess a conserved (canonical) disulfide bridge at Cys23 and Cys94, binding the CDR1 and CDR3 loops (differential to conventional VH). Another important difference between V_HH and conventional VH is the replacement in the FR2 of highly conserved hydrophobic residues Val44, Gly51, Leu52 and Trp54 - which normally participate in the interaction with the VL domain - by smaller and/or hydrophilic amino acids (mostly Phe42, Glu49, Arg50, and Gly52). These characteristics are associated with increased hydrosolubility and resistance to high temperature treatment and melt reversibility [11]. Another difference is observed in the antigen binding site. The V_HH in an HCAb acts independently from the presence of a VL chain; therefore, the antigen is recognized only by three instead of six loops. The loops in a V_HH are longer than in a VH, providing an adequately large antigen interacting surface of 600–800°A2. The sequence alignments show an enlarged variable region in the CDR1 loop and the presence of an extended CDR3 loop (Figure 3). The extended and constrained CDR loops give the molecule flexibility which promotes optimal antigen binding.

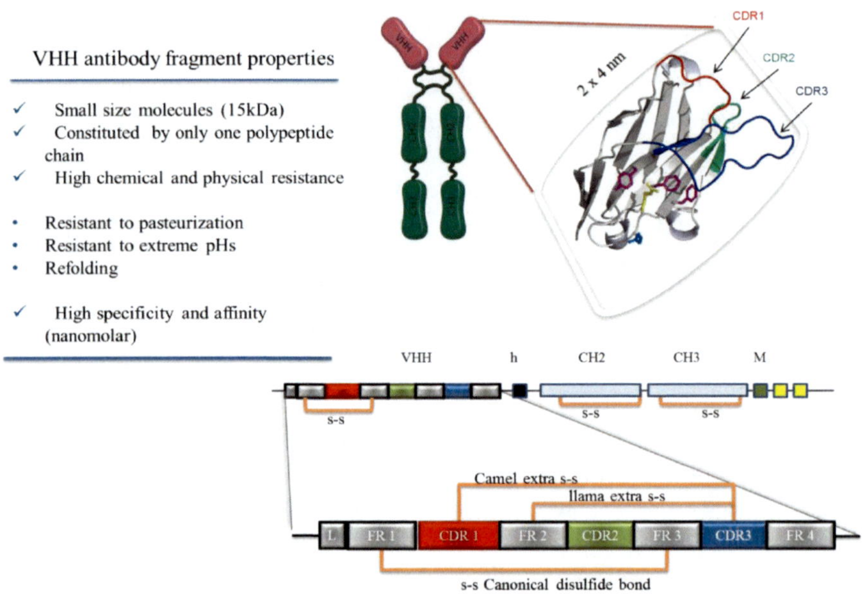

Figure 3. Schematic diagram of the V_HH domain of the camelid HCAb. H= hinge, M= transmembrane domain of membrane isoform, S-S= disulfide bond.

It is interesting to note that V_HH derived from the dromedary usually possess a long CDR3 with an average length of 18 aa and up to 23 aa. The molecules with larger CDR3 loops frequently contain an additional disulfide bond between CDR1 and CDR3, which gives more stability to the structure of the molecule. This extra bridge reduces the paratope flexibility and fixes the long CDR3 loop into an optimal conformation during antigen binding, thus, leading to a stronger affinity [12] and higher temperature resistance [11]. However, the presence of these disulfide bridges restricts camel V_HH expression to the bacteria periplasm and the yields of expression are lower than the V_HH lacking it [12]. Conversely, in V_HH derived from llamas this extra disulfide bond occurs less frequently and the CDR3 loop is on average also noticeably shorter (13 aa) than in V_HH from dromedaries. V_HH derived from llamas are similar in size to the human counterpart (VH) and possess only the canonical cystine bond resulting in structures with more flexibility than the camel antibodies and theoretically less affinity [2]. However, these llama antibodies reach higher expression yields than dromedary-derived V_HH [11].

The interloop disulfide bond in dromedary V_HH mainly occurs between the CDR1 and CDR3 loops, but it can also be found between the CDR3 and the FR2 position 50. In llama V_HH, and infrequently in dromedary V_HH as well, an interloop disulfide bond between the CDR3 loop and the CDR2 loop (position 55) is also observed.

Overall, the V_HH possess a rugby ball–shaped structure that forms a convex paratope surface. This shape is exceptionally suitable to insert in cavities on the surface of the antigen. Conversely, the paratope of conventional antibodies forms a cavity, groove, or a flat surface and these architectures have been linked to the recognition of small molecules, linear peptides, and larger antigens (such as proteins), respectively [2].

Specific Recombinant V_HH Development Strategies

The V_HH antibody fragment genes may be amplified by PCR, cloned into an expression vector and expressed as a recombinant soluble protein. Generally, specific V_HH directed to an antigen are selected from the V_HH repertoire of a camelid previously immunized with the antigen of interest. During the immunization process, affinity maturation of the antigen-specific HCAbs takes place in the animal. Then, B lymphocytes are extracted from the circulating blood and the V_HH RNA is amplified by RT-PCR. The V_HH domain is encoded by a gene fragment of only ~360 bp that can be easily PCR amplified, ligated in phage display vectors and transformed in bacteria. The DNA of the whole V_HH repertoire present in a camelid constitutes what is known as the V_HH library.

Small immune libraries of ~10^6 individual transformants are already representative of the immune V_HH repertoire of B cells present in a blood sample of ~50 ml.

Antigen-specific V_HH are selected from immune libraries by phage display or any other selection protocol, including bacterial display, yeast display, intracellular 2 hybrid selection or ribosome display.

As an example, the cloned V_HH is expressed as fusion protein with the phage coat protein pIII. Normally, two to three rounds of biopanning with the target antigen immobilized ELISA plates are sufficient to enrich the V_HH library in the desirable clones that can be further screened and selected by phage-ELISA. The obtained V_HH usually range the nanomolar to the picomolar affinities.

V_HH for Medical and Biotechnology Applications

V_HH are hydrophilic molecules, thermally stable, easy to label and have affinities in the low nanomolar to high picomolar range. Regarding biotechnological applications, V_HH are suitable to act as chaperones to crystallize challenging proteins because they lock proteins in a particular conformation, allowing their crystallization. V_HH are excellent reagents to be applied in biosensor development and protein purification [13].

Antibodies acting inside living cells are known as 'intrabodies'. V_HH fold surprisingly well into functional entities, even in the reducing intracellular environment. Therefore, intracellular expression of V_HH fused to fluorescent proteins produces useful chromobodies or fluobodies that can be used to trace their antigen in living cells [14, 15]. V_HH antibodies could become the next generation of magic bullets for immune-imaging diagnosis that can be performed as early as one hour post-injection, enabling the use of safe short live radio isotopes [16].

V_HH are suitable molecules for human therapy due to their small size (which assures optimal tissue penetration) and the poor immunogenicity (high sequence identity to human VHs). Although they are suitable for oral and topical administration, they should be humanized for systemic applications. Their small size assures a fast blood clearance in urine and different strategies have been developed to extend the serum half-life, such as fusion to other proteins, PEGilation or binding to other serum proteins [2]. V_HH for the treatment of amyloidosis, rheumatoid arthritis, cancer and against the venom of different snakes, scorpions and other poisonous animals have been developed [17]. Alternatively, V_HH can be easily fused to other molecules, such as enzymes or toxic molecules, in order to kill infected cells or tumorous cells. Finally, they are excellent tools to be used in directioning gene therapy.

Regarding infectious diseases, several V_HH have shown virus neutralizing activity. V_HH were assayed on therapeutic applications against different viruses: HIV, Hepatitis B virus, influenza virus, Respiratory Syncytial virus, Rabies virus, FMDV, Poliovirus, Rotavirus, and PERVs and dengue [10]. V_HH targeting human respiratory syncytial virus is under phase II clinical trial and shows promising results for fighting infections. Specifically for Rotavirus, two different V_HH libraries were developed and will be described in this chapter.

VP6 specific V_HH to Rotavirus

Recombinant V_HH antibody fragments are emerging as new versatile reagents for the diagnosis and also for the therapy of infectious diseases, including RV-induced diarrhea. A literature review indicated that two V_HH libraries specific to Group A Rotavirus (RVA) were generated from two immunized llamas [6, 18]. Interestingly, although the two llamas were immunized with different antigens - whole RVA particle or recombinant VP6 - finally, V_HH antibodies directed to VP6 with neutralizing activity for RVA infection were obtained in both cases. The next sections of this chapter describe the sequence from the development process of these V_HH to their testing in animal models and clinical trials in humans as a treatment for RVA diarrhea.

Target of Choice for the Development of V_HH Single Domain Antibodies to Rotavirus

The RVA VP6 inner capsid protein is highly immunogenic, constituting more than 50% of the virion mass; it has been used as the target antigen of most immunodiagnostic tests. According to the nucleotide (nt) variability (85% nt identity among VP6 of the same group), at least 17 VP6 I (for intermediate capsid shell) genotypes have been described so far; I1 and I2 are the most frequently found in human RVA strains [19]. Antibodies to VP6 were shown to cross react between different VP6 genotypes; however, most studies show that conventional Abs to VP6 lack extracellular neutralizing activity *in vitro* [20–22]. Tosser et al. developed a monoclonal Ab to VP6 (RV-133) that interacted with both double and triple-layer particles and induced partial decapsidation but failed to neutralize RVA *in vitro* [20]. Burns et al. reported two IgA monoclonal Abs to VP6 (clones 7D9 and 10C10) that did not present detectable neutralizing activity in vitro but inhibited viral transcription and completely protected against infection in vivo by intracellular neutralization during transcitosis in mice [23, 24]. Regarding the effectiveness of VP6 antibodies mediating passive protection, negative results were obtained with VP6 specific IgY in a gnotobiotic pig model of RVA infection and disease [8]. However, given the broadly reactive nature of VP6 antibodies and the special structural features of V_HH, we chose VP6 as a target protein for the development of V_HH. These V_HH molecules may show different properties from conventional antibodies and provide a broad reactive tool useful for protection from Rotavirus diarrhea as well as for the development of a diagnosis test [6]. The chosen antigen for the other Rotavirus specific V_HH library was the whole particle of RRV RVA G3P [3]. This last strategy would additionally enable the selection of V_HH antibodies specific for different RVA proteins [18].

Development of V_HH Specific Libraries to Rotavirus

The llama immunized with VP6 protein by our group of research was vaccinated intramuscularly at days 0, 21, 28, 35, and 246 with crude Sf9 cell extract containing 500 μg of recombinant VP6 protein derived from the bovine RVA C486 G6P [1] strain with the objective of obtaining V_HH antibodies highly specific to VP6 [6]. The other research group immunized a llama subcutaneously and intramuscularly at days 0, 42, 63, 97 and 153 with 5×10^{12} pfu of rhesus-monkey RVA strain RRV G3P [3] with the aim of obtaining V_HH antibodies to all the different RVA proteins [18]. Enriched lymphocyte populations were obtained from 900 ml of blood from the llama immunized with VP6 bled four days after the last immunization, and from 150 ml of blood from the llama immunized with RRV obtained on the day of the last immunization dose. Total RNA was extracted from these cells and retrotranscribed into cDNA. For V_HH library construction the V_HH genes were PCR amplified and cloned into a phagemid vector. All V_HH are encoded by a single exon with homologous sequences at both ends. Therefore, the complete *in vivo* matured V_HH repertoire of an immunized camelid can be amplified by a few sets of primers and can be cloned without major inconvenience. Although the amplification of the V_HH repertoire is simple, the method requires a strategy to avoid the cloning of VH from the conventional antibodies. The presence of VH genes in the V_HH gene library might impair subsequent pannings due to their likely sticky behavior. To get rid of the VH for the development of the anti-VP6 V_HH library (Figure 4, right panel), we first employed a pan-annealing primer that bound to a conserved region of all constant γ genes in combination with a back primer that annealed at the leader signal sequence of the VH and V_HH, so that all IgG isotypes were amplified toward their VH and V_HH end.

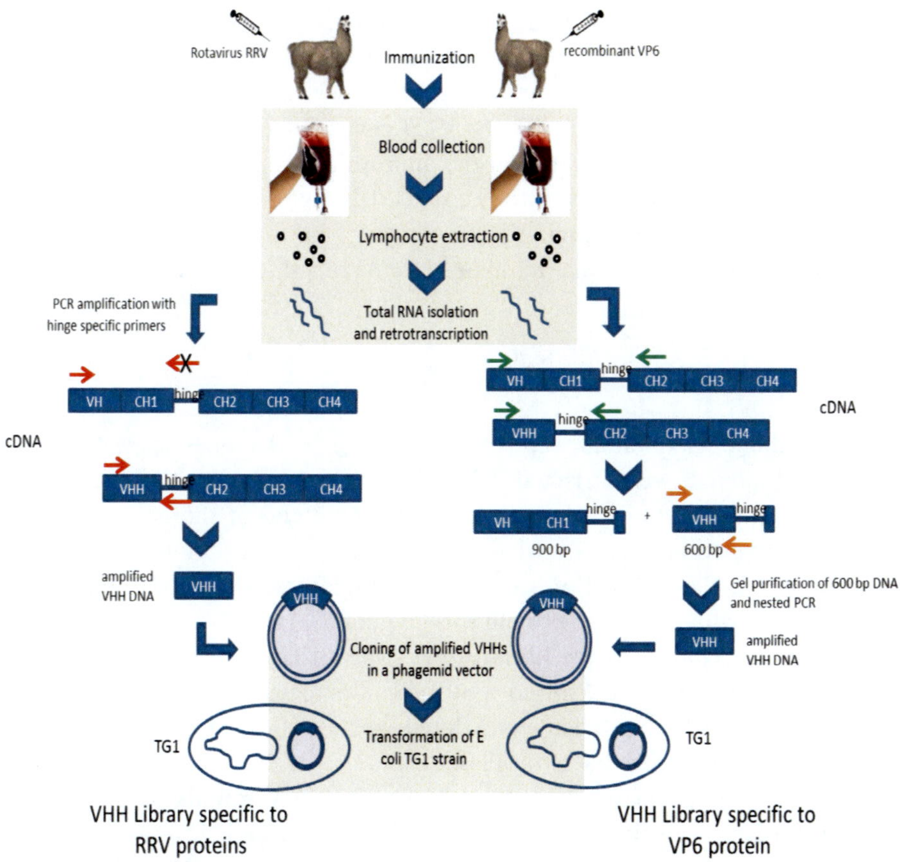

Figure 4. VHH library production strategies used for the production of anti-RVA VHH antibody fragments. On the left is a description of the strategy used by van der Vaart et al., 2006, for the production of anti RRV VHH; on the left is a depiction of the strategy used for Garaicoechea et al., 2008, for the production of VP6 specific VHH. [6, 18].

This primary PCR yields two kinds of fragments: one kind contains the CH1 exon and is derived from the heavy chain of a conventional antibody; and a second kind of fragment lacking the CH1 exon is derived from the heavy chain of the HCAb. These PCR fragments are easily separated on agarose gel and the recovery of the shorter fragment eliminates the VH sequences efficiently. A secondary PCR with nested primers annealing at the beginning and end of the V_HH is then performed to make more material and to include restriction enzyme sites for cloning purposes. The group that built the V_HH library specific to RRV RVA followed a different method previously published by van der Linden et al. [25], which makes use of PCR primers that anneal selectively on the hinge of the HCAb. This region possesses the largest sequence differences between the different isotypes, and therefore primers can be designed that will only amplify the V_HH genes (Figure 4, left panel). After cloning the amplified V_HH genes in the appropriate phage display vector, the cloned V_HH were transformed into E coli TG1 bacteria and then the two V_HH libraries were generated similarly, containing the V_HH repertoire of the lymphocytes circulating in the immunized llama blood [6, 18].

Phage Display Selection of Specific V_HH

Once the V_HH libraries were developed, the V_HH clones specific to the antigens of interest were selected using the phage display technology. In the library development the V_HH were cloned at the 3´end of the gene encoding for the pIII capsid protein of a filamentous phage, in a phagemid vector. This strategy allows the production of phages particles displaying the V_HH as a fusion protein with the phage protein pIII (Figure 5).

For the enrichment of the libraries in clones of interest several sequential rounds of panning were carried out with immobilized antigen surfaces. Antigen-bound phage particles were eluted in drastic conditions and regrown after the infection of new bacteria (Figure 5).

For the enrichment of the VP6 V_HH library, three rounds of biopanning were performed using immobilized bovine RVA IND G6P [5] as an antigen. From 192 individual clones tested after the biopanning 20 unique V_HH sequences able to bind bovine RVA IND and also the recombinant VP6 protein were obtained. Four clones showing the strongest specific binding were selected for neutralization and protection assays (2KA4, 2KD1, 3A6 and 3B2 VHH).

The selected V_HH were sub-cloned in the pHEN6 expression vector, which adds a His_6 tag to the V_HH sequence and allows the soluble expression of the V_HH in E coli periplasmic space. These V_HH were purified from the periplasmic space using affinity chromatography for His_6 tag fusion proteins [6].

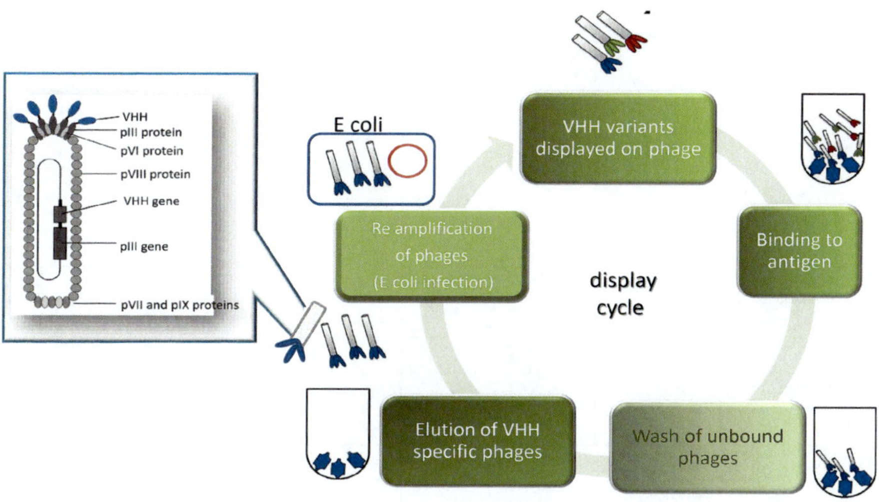

Figure 5. Structure of a phylamentous phage displaying a V_HH antibody on its surface (a) and phage display cycle (b).

For the biopanning of the RRV specific library, RRV RVA particles were captured with anti-RVA sera on immunotubes. A decreasing amount of virus and decreasing pH was used from the first to the third biopanning round to increase the astringency of the selection. After the biopanning the binding of 160 individual V_HH clones against RRV and CK RVA strains were tested and 23 unique clones that bound both strains were detected. Four clones were selected for further protection assays.

The selected V_HH were subcloned and expressed as soluble V_HH secreted to S. cerevisiae supernatant and purified using ion exchange chromatography [7] or concentrated by filtration over microcon filters with a 10 kDa cut-off [18].

Table 1. Broad reactivity of the VP6 specific V_HH antibody fragments by ELISA, Western Blot and Immmuno-EM

RVA strain	Species of origin	Genotypes	V_HH from VP6 specific library				V_HH from RRV specific library	
			ELISA results				IEM and/ or WB results	
			2KA4	2KD1	3A6	3B2	ARP1	ARP3
Gottfried	Porcine	G4-P [6]-I1	+	+	+	+		
H1	Porcine	G5-P [7]-I5	+	+	+	+		
H2	Equine	G3-P [12]-I2	+	+	+	+		
C486	Bovine	G6-P [1]-I?	+	+	+	+		
IND	Bovine	G6-P [5]-I?	+	+	+	+		
I801	Bovine	G8-P [1]-I2	+	+	+	+		
B223	Bovine	G10-P [11]-I2	+	+	+	+		
Arg720	Human	G12-P [9]-I?	+	+	+	+		
Wa	Human	G1-P [8]-I1	+	+	+	+	+	
DS-1	Human	G2-P [4]-I2	+	+	+	+	+	
SA11	Simian	G3-P [1]-I2	+	+	+	+	+	+
ST3	Human	G4-P [6]-I1	+	+	+	+	+	+
69M	Human	G8-P [10]-I2	+	+	+	+	+	+
F45	Human	G9-P [8]-I?	+	+	+	+	+	+
RRV (rivm)	Rhesus	G3-P [3]-I2					+	+
Va70	Human	G4-P [8]-I?					+	+
UP3	Human	G9-P [6]-I?					+	
CK5	Bovine						+	+

V_HH from both libraries were shown to recognize RVA strains of different species of origin and different G, P and I genotypes. Blanks mean "Not Determined".

VP6-Specific V_HH as Broadly Reactive Reagents

The usefulness of the selected V_HH against VP6 protein for RVA diagnosis was assessed using different RVA strains. The four V_HH selected from the VP6 V_HH library were able to detect all the RVA strains of human and animal origin tested, with different VP6 I-types, VP7 G and VP4 P-types (Table 1) [6, 8].

All of the V_HH selected from the library specific to RRV were able to recognize the homologous strain and the CK5 bovine RVA by ELISA [18].

Additionally, two of these V_HH were shown to bind to VP6 protein and were named ARP1or ARP3 [7]. These antibodies also proved to be broadly reactive by Immune-EM with ARP1 or ARP3 coated grids and Western Blot. ARP1 bound to cell culture adapted RVA strains and also to RVA strains of different genotypes from clinical samples (G1P [8], G2P [4], G3P [8], G4P [8], G9P [6], G9P [8], G12P [9] and G10P [11] (Table 1) [7].

These results indicate that VP6 specific binders are directed against shared epitopes and are therefore excellent and inexpensive alternatives for the use of mouse monoclonal antibodies for the design of group RVA diagnosis tests.

It was also observed that when two V_HH were fusioned, joined by a linker, to produce bivalent proteins, better reagents resulted compared to the monovalent counterpart, as capture antibodies for RVA detection by ELISA [6]

Interestingly, all the anti-VP6 V_HH antibodies recognized oligomeric forms of VP6 by Western Blot [6, 7], suggesting that they are binding to an inter-monomer interaction region; however, the exact epitopes for these V_HH have not been described.

VP6-Specific V_HH Neutralize Rotavirus *in vitro*

Most studies have shown that conventional antibodies to VP6 lack neutralizing activity [20]– [22]. However, five of the V_HH directed against VP6 showed broad neutralization against RVA strains belonging to different genotype combinations that normally do not elicit a cross-reactive neutralizing immune response [26].

Three of the five broad neutralizing V_HHs (2KD1, 3A6 and 3B2) were selected from the VP6 specific V_HH library and they completely neutralized the infectivity generated by 100 FFU of RV C486 (G6P [1]), IND (G6P [5]), B223 (G10P [11], Wa (G1P [8]), I801 (G8P [1]) and H2 (G3P [12]) strains (Table 2) [6]. V_HH 3B2 was additionally tested against many relevant RVA strains circulating in humans worldwide, including not only Wa (G1P [8]I1), but also DS1 (G2P [4]), 69M (G8P [10]), F45 (G9P [8]) and Arg720 (G12P [9]) among others (Table 2), with positive results [8]. It is interesting to note that making the V_HH bivalent impaired the neutralization capacity, suggesting it is somehow related to the molecule size [6].

Table 2. Neutralization of the infectivity of RV strains from different genotype combinations in MA104 cells

RVA strain	Species of origin	Genotypes	V_HH from VP6 specific library			V_HH from RRV specific library	
			conc. for ≥80% inhib. of FFU (μg/ml)			conc. for ≥50% inhib. of FFU (μg/ml)	
			2KD1	3A6	3B2	ARP1	AR P3
Gottfried	Porcine	G4-P [6]-I1	-	-	0.24	-	-
H1	Porcine	G5-P [7]-I5	-	-	0.98	-	-
H2	Equine	G3-P [12]-I2	3.91	15.6	3.91	-	-
C486	Bovine	G6-P [1]-I?	0.98	1.95	1.95	-	-
IND	Bovine	G6-P [5]-I?	0.98	1.95	1.95	-	-
I801	Bovine	G8-P [1]-I2	0.24	0.24	0.24	-	-
B223	Bovine	G10-P [11]-I2	0.98	7.8	0.98	-	-
Arg720	Human	G12-P [9]-I?	-	-	3.91	-	-
Wa	Human	G1-P [8]-I1	0.24	0.98	0.06	0.63*	-
DS-1	Human	G2-P [4]-I2	-	-	0.24	5.00	5.00
SA11	Simian	G3-P [1]-I2	-	-	15.63	neg*	-
ST3	Human	G4-P [6]-I1	-	-	0.98	5.00	5.00
69M	Human	G8-P [10]-I2	-	-	0.98	0.63	0.63
F45	Human	G9-P [8]-I?	-	-	0.06	0.63	0.63
RRV (rivm)	Rhesus	G3-P [3]-I2	-	-	-	2.50*	-
Va70	Human	G4-P [8]-I?	-	-	-	0.63	0.63
WI61	Human	G9-P [8]-I1	-	-	-	2.50*	-
RV4	Human	G1-P [8]-I?	-	-	-	1.25	1.25
M37	Human	G2-P [6]-I?	-	-	-	1.25	1.25
P	Human	G3-P [8]-I1	-	-	-	5.00	2.50

The neutralization was measured by the reduction in the focus fluorescent forming units (FFU) when the RVA strain was incubated with V_HH. Values labeled with a * were obtained from assays performed in CaCo cells. Dash means "Not Determined". All data were obtained from Garaicoechea et al. 2008, Vega et al. 2012 and Aladin et al. 2012 [6–8].

The other two neutralizing V_HH, ARP1 and ARP3 were selected from the RRV specific V_HH library and they neutralized the infectivity of RVA strains Wa (G1P [8]), DS-1 (G2P [4]), WI-61 (G9P [8]), 69M (G8P [10]), F45 (G9P [8]), Va70 (G4P [8]), RV4 (G1P [8]), M37 (G2P [6]), ST-3 (G4P [6]) and P(G3P [8]). ARP3 demonstrated similar neutralization activity to ARP1 (Table 2) [7].

These V_HH molecules were the first VP6 specific antibodies that showed extracellular broad neutralization of RVA infection.

Neutralization Mechanism of the VP6 V_HH

The mechanism by which V_HH antibody fragments inhibit virus replication is still unclear. Several theories have been proposed and many studies are in progress to elucidate it. The neutralizing capacity of these antibody fragments to RVA infection may be related to their small size, as bivalent V_HH antibodies showed reduced neutralizing activity compared to the monovalent counterpart. This suggests that the bivalent form, of a higher size, may have limited access to the exposed VP6 on an active triple-layered RVA particle. It was also suggested that the neutralizing V_HH may be inducing a conformational change in VP6, VP7 or VP4, impairing the interaction with a cellular receptor and preventing the binding and/or RVA entrance to the cell. Alternatively, the V_HH could be blocking virus decapsidation or the RNA transcription through occlusion of the channels of the RVA particle. It was also hypothesized that the V_HH may interfere with the secretory pathways during late replication, preventing virus assembly and release. Apart from these hypotheses, the mechanisms of VP6 V_HH neutralization and interaction with Rotavirus remain speculative and unconfirmed at this stage [5–9].

Production of VP6 Specific V_HH in Different Expression Platforms

Since VP6 specific V_HH antibody fragments showed neutralizing activity to RVA infection, they started to be considered as a potential therapy. The therapeutic concept of V_HH antibody fragments against RVA could be considered not only as a conventional drug but also as an additive to elaborate a functional food able to reduce the incidence or severity of RVA diarrhea, especially in risk populations (infants in day care centers, hospitalized children, immunosuppressed patients, etc.). Therefore, the choice of an efficient heterologous expression system, involving high production efficiency or downstream processing, would represent a step toward the clinical application of V_HH. For oral therapy a prerequisite is the elimination of any living organism that could contaminate or replicate in the intestinal tract of patients, as well as the removal of any potential contaminating toxin that may aggravate the diarrhea. The VP6 specific V_HH, genetically engineered for production, were shown to be versatile molecules and resulted as functional in the several expression platforms assayed. Specifically, the anti-VP6 V_HH have been expressed successfully in bacteria, yeast, and insect cell lines, as well as in plants such as tobacco and rice.

E coli: The four V_HH, named 2KA4, 2KD1, 3A6, and 3B2, originated from the VP6 specific V_HH library were subcloned into an expression vector (the phagemid vector pHEN6) providing an amino-terminal pELB signal to direct the expression of these proteins to the bacterial periplasmic space and a carboxy-terminal His_6 tag for further purification. The redox potential of the periplasmic environment is optimal for V_HH expression, given that it favors the correct formation of the disulfide bonds of the V_HH and a proper folding as soluble and functional proteins. After osmotic shock, the V_HH were purified from the periplasmic extract with affinity chromatography using the His_6 tag.

The yields obtained after purification at a laboratory scale (1-3 liters of bacterial culture) ranged between 20 and 50 mg of functional V_HH/liter of culture. The expression yields in *E coli* are optimal; however, exhaustive purification of the molecules is crucial for oral administration in humans. This increases the costs and makes this platform non-suitable for large-scale production [6].

S. cerevisiae: The ARP1 and ARP3 V_HH were expressed in yeast and collected from yeast supernatant. After freezing and drying the supernatant, the V_HH ARP1 represented 35% of the total mass. This platform is an excellent option for V_HH production for an oral therapy, given that no further purification is required [9].

Baculovirus system: The baculovirus expression vector system (BEVS) is a method used to efficiently produce functional recombinant proteins, including any kind of antibodies. However, the production cost of BEVS is relatively high when insect cells lines are used. An economically efficient alternative to insect cell cultures is the use of insects as living biofactories. The most used insect larvae for such purposes are the natural host of *Autographa californica*, the lepidopter *Trichoplusia ni*. Recombinant protein production by the combination of recombinant baculovirus and this insect larva has been denominated the improved baculovirus expression system (IBES®). This technology represents one of the best production alternatives based on baculovirus vectors and allows working in nonsterile conditions. These larvae provide a final product with high biosafety standards, as animal compounds are not involved in the production process and neither does cross-infection in mammals occur between pathogens infecting this lepidopter. Two constructs using the V_HH 3B2 or 2KD1 genes were generated using the IBES® technology. The encoding genes for the antibodies were cloned in phase with the mellitin signal peptide to increase productivity. For the expression of V_HH, fifth instar larvae were inoculated with a dose of 50,000 plaque forming units per larva (pfu/larva) for the 3B2 production while for 2KD1 it was 10,000 pfu/larva. The larva-derived recombinant V_HH were detected in total soluble protein (TSP) fractions obtained from infected larvae. The percentages of recombinant V_HH produced in the TSP were 2.62 and 3.63 for 2KD1 and 3B2, respectively. Recombinant V_HH were purified by affinity chromatography from the TSP and recovery rates of around 50% were achieved for both molecules. Overall, using low recombinant baculovirus doses to express the V_HH, the expression yield was 1.4 and 1.8 mg/g of insect biomass of recombinant 3B2 and 2KD1, respectively (up to 257 mg/L of insect extract). The monovalent V_HH efficiently expressed in larvae presented the same functionality as those expressed in E. coli, showing polyreactive and broad neutralizing properties against several RVA strains by ELISA and neutralization assay, respectively [27].

Transplastomic Tobacco: The main advantage of plants as bioreactors comes from the lower cost and the simplicity in scaling up. However, in order to compete against traditional expression hosts, plants must achieve a minimum accumulation of recombinant protein considered as 50 μg per gram of fresh tissue. Transplastomic plants have higher expression levels than nuclear transgenic plants, a fact attributed to the polyploidy of the chloroplast genome and the lack of silencing and position effects.

Different expression strategies were assayed in tobacco for the V_HH 3B2. One of them consisted in the expression of the V_HH in the thylakoid space. In this case, the expression levels were good. The highest accumulation of the nanobody in this V_HH transplastomic plant was observed in the oldest leaf (2–3 % TSP; 50–100 μg/g FT), highlighting its stability in the thylakoid lumen. Additionally, this V_HH presented binding activity and was able to neutralize RVA in the same way as the V_HH produced in E. coli. However, the phenotype of the plant showed growth arrest and leaf color fading when grown under normal illumination. If these plants had a normal development, the expression levels obtained would be compatible with large-scale production. This fact is essential to achieve considerable biomass in an acceptable time.

The expression of the 3B2 V_HH directly in the chloroplast stroma failed, suggesting a toxic effect of the foreign protein possibly due to incorrect folding in the environment of the stroma. The translational fusion of the protein of interest to another that presents important stability has been previously used with successful results, so in this case the V_HH was fusioned to the b-glucuronidase, a very stable protein in the chloroplast stroma, and was used as a carrier of the 3B2 V_HH. The fusion protein stabilized the V_HH expression in the stroma at high levels (3 % TSP; 70 μg/g FT) and the plants had a normal development.

However, either the fusion to the b-glucuronidase or the expression in the stroma impaired the functionality of the V_HH to recognize and neutralize RVA [28]. The expression of the VP6 specific V_HH in transplastomic plants has yet to be optimized.

Lactobodies: *Lactobacilli* are generally regarded as safe microorganisms that constitute an important component of the normal mucosal microbiota and could be administered orally as a food product. Many strains of *lactobacilli* show probiotic properties and have been successfully used for intervention against RVA diarrhea [29]. In the context of the development of a therapy against RVA diarrhea, the VP6 specific V_HH antibody ARP1 was expressed by *lactobacilli* for the *in situ* delivery of this molecule. The V_HH was expressed, either anchored to the surface of the *lactobacillus* or as a soluble protein. For the generation of the surface-expressed V_HH, the DNA fragment coding for ARP1–E-tag (E-tagged for detection and purification) was cloned upstream of the DNA encoding for an anchor sequence of the *Lactobacillus* P protein in the expression vector pLP501. Then the ARP1-E V_HH was expressed as a fusion protein with the last 244 aa of the proteinase P protein of *Lactobacillus casei* [30, 31]. To generate the secreted ARP1-E antibody fragment, a stop codon (TAA) was inserted at the 3´end of the E-tag and also cloned into the vector pLP501. Transformation of *L. paracasei* was performed and modified *lactobacilli* were obtained [32].

The expression of soluble ARP1-E V_HH by *lactobacilli* was successfully detected by ELISA while the expression of ARP1-anchored *lactobacilli* was detected by immunofluorescence of the transformant *lactobacilli* with anti-E tag antibody. Furthermore, the presence of live *lactobacilli*, which express the anchored V_HH, was detected in the jejunum and ilium of mice 48 hours after the oral administration of $1x10^8$ cfu, while at 96 hours it was no longer detectable.

Affinity-purified ARP1 from the supernatant of *lactobacilli* secreting the V_HH could neutralize 80% of the infectivity of RVA relative to a control V_HH at a concentration of 125 ng/ml, while ARP1-anchored lactobacilli could also effectively neutralize RVA in a dose-dependent manner, starting at 1000 bacteria/well. When the anchored construct was used, the numerous antibody fragments expressed on the bacterial surface resulted in the formation of "biological beads" that allowed high-avidity binding due to multivalency and thus, promoted strong agglutination and subsequent clearance of the virus. Pant et al. suggested that this multivalent display of ARP1 on *lactobacilli* caused neutralization by aggregation [32].

Thinking of a therapy directed to a single epitope has limitations regarding the selection of resistant mutants and cross-reactivity to the circulating or new genotypes of virus, and typically requires high amounts of antibodies for neutralization. Two anti VP6 V_HH from the RRV V_HH library - ARP1 and ARP3 - were shown to bind to different epitopes. These two V_HH antibodies were produced as bivalent and bispecific constructs on the surface of *lactobacilli*.

Bivalent ARPs (ARP1–ARP1, ARP3–ARP3, ARP1–ARP3 or ARP3–ARP1) were generated by fusing the two fragment encoding genes, end to end (without a linker), using PCR [33]. The genes encoding the monomeric and bivalent ARPs were amplified and cloned between NcoI and NotI restriction sites into the pAF900 plasmid [34]. In this vector, gene expression is under the control of the aggregation promoting factor (apf) gene promoter of Lactobacillus crispatus M247. The vector contains the signal peptide of the apf gene to mediate protein secretion, an E-tag encoding gene and an anchor sequence (the last 231 amino acids of the proteinase P protein of *L. paracasei*) for surface display. Transformation of *L. paracasei* was performed.

The expression of V_HH constructs display on the lactobacilli surface as well as the ability of these V_HH to bind RRV RVA was proven by flow cytometry. The ARP3–ARP1- producing *lactobacilli* displayed the fusion proteins in high levels and was the construct that showed the stronger binding to RVA (RRV; 3.5-fold higher geometric mean over monovalent *lactobacilli*-produced ARP1) and was the best binder among all the constructs tested. *Lactobacilli* producing bispecific ARP3–ARP1 showed neutralizing activity of RRV infection *in vitro*, while wild-type *L. paracasei* did not neutralize the RRV RVA infection [33].

The advantages of using genetically modified *lactobacilli* include cost-efficient production, a long shelf-life when they are lyophilized, simple logistics for distribution, and ease of administration.

In situ production of V_HH antibody fragments locally in the gastrointestinal tract of the host not only reduces the cost of purification but also circumvents the practical problem of the degradation of orally administered antibodies in the stomach. The soluble V_HH expressed in lactobacilli as well as the lactobacilli displaying the different V_HH were assayed in a suckling mice model for protection against RVA infection and diarrhea.

Rice: The expression of the VP6 specific V_HH protein in transgenic rice may lead to the development of a rice-based, orally administered product against RVA. Antibody-producing tobacco leaves need storage under–20 degrees, and antibody-producing tomatoes need a temperature below 4 degrees. In contrast, antibody-producing cereals such as rice and wheat, as well as pea seeds, can be stored at room temperature. The rice powder or rice water may constitute novel approaches to prevent or treat RVA diarrhea and may be used in both developed and developing countries, as a complement to the current vaccine and in situations where live attenuated vaccines are contraindicated.

Using a binary vector (pZH2Bik45G1B), a codon-optimized ARP1 gene combined with a RNAi suppression cassette was transfected into rice plants (Nippon-Bare) using Agrobacterium tumefaciens–mediated transformation (Figure 6). The expression of the prolamin (13 kDa) and glutelin (22–23 kDa and 34–37 kDa) was suppressed by the RNAi and the 12 kDa V_HH protein was predominantly expressed in the transgenic rice. ARP1 is water soluble, so it was released from the rice powder after PBS dilution (rice water) [5].

The yield of soluble ARP1 (95% of the ARP1 total yield) was an average of 170 μg per rice seed, representing 11.9% of the total seed protein (0.85% of seed weight) and the expression was shown to occur throughout the entire seed. In contrast, transgenic rice, without RNAi suppression of prolamin and glutelin, yielded only 14 μg of ARP1/seed.

Proteins of WT rice seeds generally accumulate into 2 different types of protein bodies (PB), PB-I contain prolamin as the major component and is resistant to digestive enzymes, whereas PB-II contains mainly glutelin and is easily digested in the gut. When the sections were examined by immune electron microscopy, ARP1 was predominantly localized in PB-II and the cytoplasm between PB-I and PB-II.

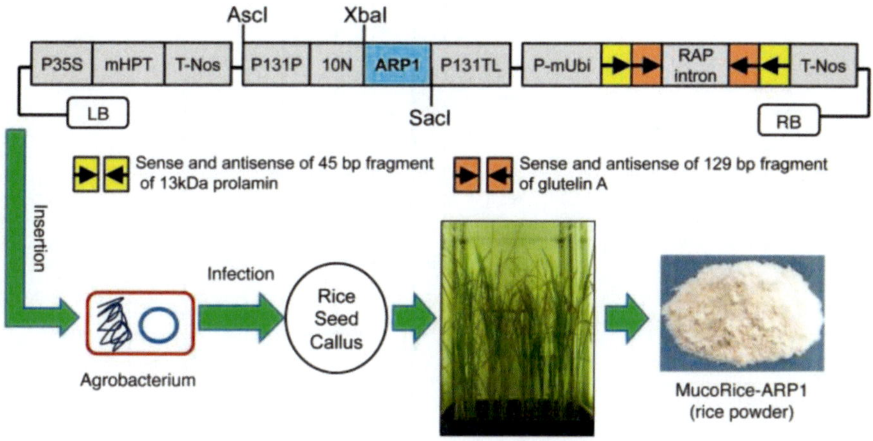

J Clin Invest. Sep 3, 2013; 123(9):3829-3838. Copyright© 2013, American Society for Clinical Investigation.

Figure 6. Expression and localization of water-soluble ARP1 in transgenic rice. Inserted plasmid for overexpression of ARP1 in rice seeds. P35S, CaMV35S promoter; mHPT, modified hygromycin phosphotransferase; P131P, 13-kDa prolamin promoter; 10N, signal sequence of 10-kDa prolamin; P131TL, 13-kDa prolamin terminator; T-Nos, nos terminator; RAP intron, rice aspartic protease intron; P-mUbi, ubiquitin promoter; LB, T-DNA left border; RB, T-DNA right border.

The V_HH expressed in rice showed a similar binding to rhesus RVA (RRV) compared to yeast-derived ARP1 and showed resistance to heat treatment of 30 min at 100°C (67% of remaining binding activity by ELISA of rice water with ARP1). Additionally, when the rice was stored at room temperature for more than 1 year, the neutralizing activity of the derived rice water remained intact compared to that of freshly harvested ARP1-rice.

Rice water containing the rice-expressed ARP1 was able to neutralize the human RVA strains 69M (G8P [10]), F45 (G9P [8]) and Va70 (G4P [8]) using the same dose of rice-expressed ARP1 as purified yeast derived ARP1 (1.25 µg /ml). For the RVA strains Wa (G1P [8]), ST-3 (G4P [6]), 4 times the amount of rice water of Rice-ARP1(10 µg/ml) was needed compared to purified yeast-derived ARP1 [5].

Table 3. Summary of the experiments performed in the mouse model

V_HH	Source	V_HH dose	Challenge strain	Challenge dose	Challenge day	Nº mice/ group	Max Diarrhea %	Diarrhea onset (day from start of experiment)	Virus shedding	Reference
3B2	Purified from E coli	100 µg/daily day 0-4	C486	6 x 10^5 FFU (30 DD50/100 µl)	1 (2 hs post VHH doses)	15	39*	2	N/D	Garaicoechea et al., 2008
2KD1							73			
non rel							100			
3B2	Purified from E coli	100 µg/daily day 0-4	ECw	300 DD50/100 µl	1 (2 hs post VHH doses)	10	40*	3	100% day 5	
2KD1							40*	5	0%* day 5	
non rel							100	5	100% day 5	
3B2	Purified from insect larvae	100 µg/daily day 0-4	ECw	300 DD50/100 µl	1 (2 hs post VHH doses)	17	47*	3	47%* day 5	Silvia Gomez-Sebastián et al., 2012
2KD1						18	59		6%* day 5	
3B2 + 2KD1		50 µg+50µg/ daily day 0-4				10	40*		30%* day 5	
3B2	TSP from larvae	100 µg VHH/ daily day 0-4	ECw			12	50		33%* day 5	
2KD1						12	50		8%* day 5	
-		-				12	100		100% day 5	
ARP1	Expressed in S. cerevicae	2 x 10µg/10µl/ daily day 0-4	RRV	2 x 10^7 UFF/10 µl (20 DD50)	1 (pre-mix RRV with VHH)	6	33	2	N/D	van der Vaart, 2006
-	-	-			1	8	100			

V_HH	Source	V_HH dose	Challenge strain	Challenge dose	Challenge day	Nº mice/ group	Max Diarrhea %	Diarrhea onset (day of the experiment)	Virus shedding	Reference
ARP1	Expressed in S. cerevicae	5µg/10µl/daily day 0-4	RRV	2 x 10^7 UFF/10 µl (20 DD50)	1 (2 hs prior to VHH dose)	9	~90	2	N/D	van der Vaart, 2006
		20µg/10µl/daily day 0-4				8	~100			
		50µg/10µl/daily day 0-4				10	~70			
		100µg/10µl/daily day 0-4				9	~40			
-	-	-				8	~100			
ARP1	Expressed in S. cerevicae	10µg/10 µl/daily day 0-4	RRV	2 x 10^7 UFF/10 µl (20 DD50)	1 (2 hs post VHH dose)	8	38*	3		Pant et al., 2011
ARP3						7	43*			
ARP1+ ARP3		5µg+5µg/10 µl/daily day 0-4				8	12*			
-	-	-				8	100			
Biv ARP1-ARP1	Anchored to L.paracasei	1 x 10^8 cfu/10 µl/ daily day 0-4	RRV	2 x 107 UFF/10 µl (20 DD50)	1 (2 hs post VHH dose)	14	~72	3		
Biv ARP3-ARP3						14	~60*			
BivARP3-ARP1						12	33*		a# 4.1 x 10^1 copies 4 dpc	
ARP1						7	~42*		a# 4.3 x 10^1 copies 4 dpc	

Table 3. (Continued)

V_HH	Source	V_HH dose	Challenge strain	Challenge dose	Challenge day	Nº mice/ group	Max Diarrhea %	Diarrhea onset (day from start of experiment)	Virus shedding	Reference
ARP3	Anchored to L.paracasei	1 x 10^8 cfu/10 µl/ daily day 0-4	RRV	2 x 10^7 UFF/10 µl (20 DD50)	1 (2 hs post VHH dose)	7	~60*	3		Pant et al., 2011
ARP3 + ARP1						7	~42*	2		
-	-	-				12	~100	3	a 2.1 x 10^3 copies 4 dpc	
ARP1	Purified from S. cerevicae	10 µl/daily day 0-3	RRV	2 x 10^7 UFF/10 µl (20 DD50)	0 (2 hs prior to VHH dose)	7	43	2		
ARP3						5	~60			
ARP1+ ARP3						6	~35			
-	-	-				6	~85			
BivARP3-ARP1	Anchored to L.paracasei	1 x 108 cfu/10 µl/ daily day 0-3				7	~60		a 3.1 x 10^3 copies 4 dpc	
ARP1						8	~60			
ARP3						8	~100			
non rel						7	~80			
-	-	-				5	~100			

V_HH	Source	V_HH dose	Challenge strain	Challenge dose	Challenge day	Nº mice/ group	Max Diarrhea %	Diarrhea onset (day of the experiment)	Virus shedding	Reference
ARP1	Anchored to L.paracasei	1 x 10^8 cfu/10 µl/ daily day 0-4	RRV	2 x 10^7 UFF/10 µl (20 DD50)	1 (2 hs post VHH dose)	27	~40*	2	57% day 4	Pant et al., 2006
	Secreted by L.Paracasei					10	~65*	2	N/D	
-	L. paracasei	-	RRV	2 x 10^7 UFF/10 µl (20 DD50)	1 (2 hs post VHH dose)	17	~65*	2	N/D	Pant et al., 2006
-	-						100		83% 3 dpc	
ARP1	Anchored to L.paracasei	1 x 10^8 cfu/10 µl/ daily day 0-4	RRV	4 x 10^6 UFF/10 µl (4 DD50)	1 (2 hs post VHH dose)		6	2	0% 2 dpc	
-	L. paracasei						50	2	100% 2 dpc	
ARP1	Water Rice	2 x 8.5 µg/daily day 0-3	RRV	2 x 10^7 UFF/10 µl (20 DD50)	0 (9 hs post VHH dose)	6 to 10	~35	2	~1x 10^3 copies 3 dpc	Daisuke Tokuhara et al., 2014
ARP1	in Water Rice, 30 min 100ºC						~50	2		
-	Water Rice	2 doses/daily day 0-3					~100	2	~1x 10^5 copies 3 dpc	

Table 3. (Continued)

V_HH	Source	V_HH dose	Challenge strain	Challenge dose	Challenge day	N° mice/ group	Max Diarrhea %	Diarrhea onset (day from start of experiment)	Virus shedding	Reference
ARP1	Water Rice	2 x 8.5 µg/daily day 0-3	RRV	2 x 10^7 UFF/10 µl (20 DD50)	0 (9 hs post VHH dose)	6 to 10	~20	2		Daisuke Tokuhara et al., 2014
ARP1	in Water Rice, rice ≥ 1 year						~35	2		
-	PBS	2 doses/daily day 0-3					~85	2		
ARP1	Water Rice	2 x 8.5 µg/daily day 0-3	RRV	2 x 10^7 UFF/10 µl (20 DD50)	0 (9 hs prior to VHH dose)	6 to 10	~35	2		
-	Water Rice	2 doses/daily day 0-3					~100	2		

TSP: Tissue Soluble Protein

[#] Statistically significantly different from the control untreated group, percentage with diarrhea (Fisher exact test, p<0,05).

[*] Statistically significantly different from the control untreated group, percentage with diarrhea (Kruskal-Wallis non parametric rank sum test, p ≤0.05)

[a] RNA copies/mg small intestine

dpc: days post challenge.

Non rel: non related V_HH

VP6 Specific V_HH as Protection against RVA Induced Diarrhea and Infection

Evaluation of the Protective Capacity against Diarrhea and Virus Shedding of the VP6-Specific V_HH in a Suckling Mice Model

After proving the neutralizing activity *in vitro* of the anti VP6 V_HH, several neonatal mouse model experiments were designed and carried out by different research groups. The results are summarized in Table 3.

Purified V_HH expressed in E. coli: The prophylactic effect of monovalent V_HH originated from the VP6 specific V_HH library was also evaluated in a neonatal mouse model. In this case, pups received a single intragastric dose of 100 μg of V_HH daily for 5 days (day 0 to day 4) and were challenged on day 1 not only with the homologous virus to the antigen used in the vaccination (BRV C486) but also with a murine RV ECw. The challenge with RVA was performed by the intragastric route to ensure that all of the inoculum was received by the pup. The intragastric administration of 100 μg daily of the V_HH 3B2 induced partial protection against RVA-induced diarrhea caused by both BRV C486 and by a highly infectious murine RVA ECw in a neonatal mouse model. Furthermore, for mice treated with V_HH 3B2 and challenged with murine EC RVA, there was a delay of 2 days in the onset of diarrhea compared to the non-treated group, and 96 hs post-challenge a significant decrease in virus shedding was observed in the mice intestine homogenates compared to the non-treated group. In the group treated with the monovalent V_HH 2KD1, only 27% of the pups were protected against diarrhea caused by BRV C486. However, after challenge with the ECw murine strain, 60% of the pups were protected, and no virus was detected in the intestine homogenates at 96 h post-challenge [6]. This observation is in agreement with the high neutralization capacity of this V_HH. As murine RV ECw spread in littermates, cases of diarrhea that developed 24 h later or more after the first case in a litter could not be due to the initial inoculum and therefore were not considered. Pups were euthanized at 96 h post-inoculation, given that the peak of intestinal virus shedding in suckling mice was reported to be at that point [35]. Similar results were obtained in the suckling mouse model with the VP6 specific V_HH expressed in larvae using the Baculovirus system [27].

Purified V_HH expressed in yeast: The V_HH originated from the RRV V_HH library were evaluated in a suckling mice model challenged with heterologous

RVA RRV. One of these V_HH showed protective capacity. In one of the experiments, it was observed that if, prior to administration to the pups, the challenge RVA RRV inoculum was mixed with the V_HH, 20 μg of V_HH ARP1 administered daily were enough to reduce the mean number of diarrhea days to 0.33±0.21 ($p = 0.0007$) compared to 2.87±0.29 days for untreated mice. The number of pups with diarrhea was significantly lower at day 2 in the treated group compared to the untreated group. Moreover, at days 3, 4 and 5 none of the pups in the ARP1 treated group displayed signs of diarrhea compared to the majority of the pups in the other RRV treated groups. However, when the challenge inoculum was administered separately from the V_HH, higher amounts of V_HH (100 μg of V_HH administered daily) were necessary to reach similar results of around 60% of mice protected from diarrhea [18]. The ARP1 fragment selected reacted with a variety of human strains, but showed very limited cross-reactivity with the murine EDIM RVA strain, as tested by ELISA. For that reason, the murine RVA was not used for the challenge and RRV was chosen for the development of the mouse-infection model.

Later, Pant et al. tested the additive effect of the combination of V_HH ARP1 with V_HH ARP3. That study showed that ARP1 and ARP3 administered to the pups individually protected from diarrhea in 62 and 57%, respectively; however, when the V_HH were combined an additive effect was observed and 88% of the pups were protected from RVA diarrhea [33].

The V_HH that showed protection from RVA diarrhea in van der Vaart's publication [18] is the same that was tested by Pant et al. 2011 [33]. In both experiments, the same V_HH (ARP1) was expressed in S. cerevisae and the mice experiments were performed similarly, with some small differences between them. In the study by van der Vaart et al., the challenge was performed on day 1, two hours prior to the 2nd dose of V_HH, while Pant et al. performed the challenge two hours after the 2nd dose of V_HH (or two hours prior to the 1st dose). While in Pant et al.'s 2011 study, 10 μg of V_HH ARP1 protected 62% of mice from diarrhea induced with 20 DD50 of RRV (challenge performed 2 hs prior to the 2nd dose), in van der Vaart et al.'s study a dose of 10 μg/day of V_HH ARP1 did not protect any pup from diarrhea (100% diarrhea) and 100 μg of ARP1/day were necessary to achieve a protection of around 60%. These results highlight the limitations of the mouse model robustness and emphasize that small differences in the design of the experiment could lead to different conclusions.

V_HH expressed in lactobacilli: The prophylactic effect of transformed *lactobacilli* was tested using a single oral inoculum of 20 DD50 of RRV on

day 1. A 10^8 cfu dose of *lactobacilli* was orally administered to each pup once daily, starting on day 0 and continuing until day 4. The prevalence of diarrhea was significantly lower in mice treated with ARP1-anchored *lactobacilli*, compared with that in untreated mice or that in mice treated with irrelevant V_HH-anchored *lactobacilli*. In addition, ARP1-anchored *lactobacilli* significantly reduced the duration and the severity score (~50%), compared with that in untreated mice or those treated with irrelevant V_HH-anchored *lactobacilli*. The ARP1-secreting *lactobacilli* did not confer protection against RVA induced diarrhea, possibly due to the low levels of secretion of soluble V_HH.

On day 4 after infection, the virus load in the intestines of mice that received ARP1-anchored *lactobacilli* was significantly lower than that of mice given *lactobacilli* expressing an irrelevant anchored V_HH according to the VP7 Real Time PCR results. RVA was not detectable in 43% of the group that received ARP1-anchored *lactobacilli*, or in 17% of the untreated group.

The prophylactic potential of the ARP1-anchored *lactobacilli* for prevention of infection and diarrhea in mice challenged with only 4 DD50 of RRV was analyzed. The pups inoculated with RRV developed diarrhea and at day 2 after infection the diarrhea prevalence was 50%, compared with 6% in the group treated with ARP1-anchored bacteria. Intestinal sections collected from the distal ileum of mice were also analyzed for virus load by real-time PCR. None of the mice treated with ARP1-anchored *lactobacilli* had any detectable virus on day 3, while the virus was detected in the untreated group [32].

Bivalent ARP3-ARP1 anchored to *L. paracasei* demonstrated 67% protection against diarrhea and significantly reduced virus load in a prophylactic experiment. However, when the same V_HH expressing *lactobacilli* were administered two hours after challenge, the protection rate was reduced to 45% and no difference was observed in virus load compared to the untreated control (Table 3) [33].

Rice-V_HH: All 4-day-old mice infected with RRV and given PBS or WT rice developed diarrhea. When Rice-ARP1 (containing 8.5 μg of ARP1) was prophylactically given to neonatal mice twice a day for 4 days, the percentage of animals with diarrhea on day 2 after RRV inoculation was 35%, significantly lower than in mice receiving PBS or WT rice (100% diarrhea). Heat-treated Rice-ARP1 for 30 minutes at 94°C used prophylactically against RRV-induced diarrhea also significantly reduced the percentage of animals with diarrhea on day 2 in comparison with mice receiving PBS or WT rice. No significant difference was observed between heat-treated and non–heat-treated

Rice-ARP1 in their ability to reduce the percentage of mice with diarrhea and disease severity (non-heat-treated 35% versus heat-treated 50%). Long-term (>1 year) stored Rice-ARP1 applied prophylactically (8.5 μg of ARP1, 9 hs prior to challenge and then twice a day) significantly reduced the incidence of diarrhea and disease severity compared to that of mice receiving PBS and was as effective as freshly harvested Rice-ARP1 (35% diarrhea for stored rice versus 20% diarrhea for fresh rice).

Rice-ARP1 was also given therapeutically (8.5 μg of ARP1, 9 hours after RRV challenge and then twice a day); the percentage of mice with the virus induced diarrhea was also significantly lower than in the control mice receiving PBS or WT rice (35% versus 100%).

The virus load in the intestines of RRV-inoculated mice that received MucoRice-ARP1 was significantly reduced compared with that of mice given PBS ($n = 6$, $P = 0.002$) or WT rice ($P < 0.01$)($n = 6$, $P = 0.002$). Intragastrically administered Rice-ARP1 containing rice water (8.5 μg of solubleARP1) was detected in the small intestine of the mice (4 days after birth) for at least 6 hours. In some mice (40%, $n = 5$), MucoRice-ARP1 could be detected even 9 hours after intragastric administration [5].

VP6 Specific V_HH 3B2 Protect Gnotobiotic Pigs from RVA Induced Diarrhea

The VP6 specific V_HH 3B2, originated from the VP6 vaccinated llama, was shown to possess broad neutralizing activity *in vitro* and protected suckling mice against RVA induced diarrhea. These results led us to design a pre-clinical study in the Rotavirus gnotobiotic (Gn) pig model to evaluate the ability of this V_HH to protect piglets experimentally challenged with one of the most prevalent strains of human RVA, Wa G1P [8], from virus induced diarrhea and shedding [8]. The neonatal Gn pig model was chosen because Gn piglets are a widely known animal model susceptible to human RVA infection and disease and the pathogenicity of RVA in Gn piglets mimics that of natural RVA infection in infants. Furthermore, their gastrointestinal physiology and mucosal immune system resemble those of human infants [36, 37].

The V_HH was scaled up in the Improved Baculovirus Expression System (IBES technology), which uses baculovirus expression vectors in combination with Trichoplusia ni larvae as living biofactories. The expression and functional evaluation of the V_HH expressed in this platform were previously described in this chapter.

According to the experimental design Gn pigs received 210 ml twice a day of milk supplemented with the different passive treatments from the first day of life and for the following 8 days. At 72 hours of age, the pigs were challenged with $10^{6.7}$ FFU of RVA Wa.

The 3B2 V_HH clone expressed in insect larvae protected 100% of the treated animals from RVA-induced diarrhea when administered daily as a milk supplement at a final Wa RVA ELISA Ab titer of 4096 (VN titer of 256), which corresponds to around 44 mg of V_HH/day or 20–40 mg/kg/day (in the suckling mice model, the amount of V_HH administered was 22.2 mg/kg/day). Although the Gn pigs were protected against diarrhea, the virus shedding was detected in all animals in the V_HH group (5 out of 5 infected animals). Although the mean onset of virus shedding was similar in all groups of pigs, in the V_HH group the mean duration (3.0 days; p= 0.0012) and the AUC (6.16104 FFU/ml*day; p= 0.0055) were significantly lower than the ones in the non-treated group (mean duration: 5.6 days, AUC: 1.86106 FFU/ml*day).

The administration of control *larvae* as passive treatment (CL) failed to prevent RVA-associated diarrhea and did not significantly modify piglets' immune responses to Wa human RVA, but showed a trend toward less severe diarrhea, virus shedding and a lower number of ASC compared to the non-treated group [8].

Passive or active protection against RVA diarrhea is the most desirable outcome of any treatment or vaccination and can be achieved even when continued viral shedding is detected in stools. Moreover, the asymptomatic infection allows development of active immunity to prevent subsequent natural RVA infections.

Serum, coproAbs, and ASC responses were tested to assess the development of the pigs' immune responses to Wa RVA. The highest ASC responses to Wa RVA were in the GALT at 21 days post-inoculation, with lower ASC numbers in systemic lymphoid tissues. Our results indicate that pigs receiving passive Ab treatment with V_HH had the same isotype profile of IgA ASC but of lower magnitude than piglets in the non-treated group, thus suggesting some interference effect. A short delay in the development of the immune response and a lower number of ASC were also evident in the group of pigs treated with V_HH (in particular, reduced IgA ASC in the jejunum).

However, the magnitude of the Ab responses developed was potent enough to prevent Wa RVA diarrhea after a second exposure to the virus, in agreement with previous reports [38].

It is well documented that under physiological, non-inflamed conditions, dendritic cells migrate from mucosa to present antigens in the lymph nodes. As a result, dietary antigens are presented in association with signals that drive a suppressive immune response. The oral administration of V_HH 3B2 might induce a tolerant state, thereby preventing the host from eliciting an anti-V_HH immune response. However, further studies must first be conducted to confirm this statement.

Equally important, no heterologous Abs derived from the V_HH were detected in sera of treated animals, which suggests that there was no transmission of V_HH from the gut lumen into the blood. In summary, our findings show the potential value of broad neutralizing VP6-specific V_HH antibody fragments as a treatment that might complement the use of serotype-specific RVA vaccines.

VP6 Specific V_HH ARP1 in Clinical Trial with Human Infants

Prior to the field trial, the safety of the rehydrated yeast powder containing ARP1 V_HH was assessed in healthy adults and children. Then, a double-blind placebo-controlled trial was carried out at Dhaka Hospital, Bangladesh with 176 male infants (6-24 months old) with severe RVA associated diarrhea to test the efficacy of the anti VP6 V_HH ARP1 as a treatment for this condition. The infants were randomly given a fixed oral dose of ARP1 (n = 88) or placebo (maltodextrin, n=88) for a maximum of 5 days. The ARP preparation consisted of a freeze-dried yeast supernatant composed of approximately 35% ARP1, 30% yeast cell protein and peptides, 30% sugars and a small amount of other components including salts and minerals.

To administer the ARP1, individual sachets containing 165 mg of the ARP preparation, 835 mg maltodextrin (Glucidex IT12, Roquette, France), and 5 mg caramel color no. 663 (D. D. Williamson & Co., Louisville, KY) were utilized. As the actual body weights ranged from 5.69 to 11.29 kg, the administration of three sachets per day resulted in an actual dose of 15−30 mg ARP1 per kg body weight per day. The placebo consisted of 1000 mg of maltodextrin with 5 mg caramel color. Each dose was resuspended in 10 mL oral rehydrating solution and administered orally by the nursing staff at the hospital. Treatments were administered for a minimum of 4 days (if the diarrhea resolved) and a maximum of 5 days.

In both the treatment and placebo groups, 85 children completed the study. Fifty adverse events were reported during the intervention period (29 in active treatment, 21 in placebo) and 28 events were reported at follow-up (up to day 21). Based on the overall frequencies of occurrence of these events in the 2 treatment groups, no events related to the intake of ARP1 were detected. As such, no safety concerns were identified in this study.

In the treatment group, 26 children had concomitant infections (29%), while 24 (28%) had concomitant infections in the placebo group. For the correct evaluation of ARP1 as oral therapy only children with and exclusive RVA infection were considered. When an exclusive RVA infection was present, the total cumulative stool output in the placebo group was 305.47 g/kg body weight (n = 63). In the parallel ARP1 group, it was 237.03 g/kg body weight (n = 61), which represents a significant difference in stool output of 68.44 g/kg body weight (95% confidence interval [CI]: 18.27−118.59; P = .0079) and an overall reduction of 22.5%.

Table 4. Effect of Intervention on Stool Output in Subjects with Exclusive Rotavirus Infection

Day of study	Stool volume, g/kg, mean ± SD		
	ARP1 (n=59)	Placebo (n=61)	P value
1	79.7 ±38.6	91.9 ±35.5	0.07
2	69.0 ±38.7	86.1 ±44.0	0.03
3	56.2 ±36.6	75.9 ±51.3	0.02
4	42.1 ±33.5	62.5 ±53.4	0.01
5*	34.2 ±26.9	60.5 ±50.2	0.01

SD: standard deviation.
P value of Student´s t test.
*n= 37 (treated group); n=38 (placebo group).

There were no differences in total stool output when concomitant infections were present or when the groups were assessed together. ARP1 treatment in patients with exclusive Rotavirus infection resulted in significant reductions in stool output on days 2−5 in comparison with placebo.

To examine the change in the stool output rate more thoroughly, the linear mixed effect model was applied to assess the datasets. The model was based on the intention to treat the population with exclusive RVAs infection and used observations from the first four days of intervention. In the placebo group, stool output reduced at a rate of 9.13 g/kg/d (95% CI: 6.37−11.89). In the ARP1 group, stool output reduced at a rate of 14.70 g/kg/d, which is an additional 5.57 g/kg/d (95% CI: 2.07−9.07) in comparison with the placebo group. This change in the rate of stool output was significantly different from the placebo group (P = .002), and represents a 61% reduction in comparison [9].

The effect of the active treatment on diarrhea duration was not significantly different from the placebo group and no significant differences in duration of viral clearance were found between the active and placebo groups by ELISA. This clinical trial is registered with clinicaltrials.gov, number NCT01259765 (http://clinicaltrials.gov/show/NCT01259765).

The stool output is the key outcome measure for pediatric anti-diarrheal medications. Many studies on other anti-RVA associated diarrhea treatments, such as the anti-diarrheal drug nitrazoxanide, root extract of Potentilla tormentilla, zinc supplementation, or probiotic supplementation, have shown some benefits from these treatments for RVA associated gastroenteritis; however, no effect was observed on stool output and no data was given on that parameter. In placebo-controlled clinical trials in which stool output was reported, racecadotril, diosmectite, and immunoglobulins have all shown success in reducing stool output by approximately 40%–50% in the treatment groups [9].

In terms of clinical implications, the improvement in the rate of reduction of stool output through this V_HH treatment is encouraging. The V_HH ARP1 used in the treatment of RVA-induced diarrhea in male infants could be beneficial in terms of case management. Based on the current findings, optimized studies should now be designed to fully determine the overall efficacy of this V_HH toward RVA-induced diarrhea in infants in general. Such studies should be longitudinal, and multicenter in nature, in order to fully assess the clinical relevance of this anti RVA V_HH.

References

[1] Hamers-Casterman, C; Atarhouch, T; Muyldermans, S; Robinson, G; Hamers, C; Songa, EB; Bendahman, N; Hamers, R. "Naturally occurring antibodies devoid of light chains.," *Nature*, vol. 363, 446–448, 1993.

[2] Muyldermans, S. "Nanobodies: natural single-domain antibodies.," *Annu. Rev. Biochem.*, vol. 82, no. March, 775–97, Jan. 2013.

[3] Flajnik, MF; Deschacht, N; Muyldermans, S. "A case of convergence: Why did a simple alternative to canonical antibodies arise in Sharks and Camels?," *PLoS Biol.*, vol. 9, 2011.

[4] Wesolowski, J; Alzogaray, V; Reyelt, J; Unger, M; Juarez, K; Urrutia, M; Cauerhff, A; Danquah, W; Rissiek, B; Scheuplein, F; Schwarz, N; Adriouch, S; Boyer, O; Seman, M; Licea, A; Serreze, DV; Goldbaum, FA; Haag, F; Koch-Nolte, F. "Single domain antibodies: Promising experimental and therapeutic tools in infection and immunity," *Medical Microbiology and Immunology*, vol. 198. 157–174, 2009.

[5] Tokuhara, D; Álvarez, B; Mejima, M; Hiroiwa, T; Takahashi, Y; Kurokawa, S; Kuroda, M; Oyama, M; Kozuka-hata, H; Nochi, T; Sagara, H; Aladin, F; Marcotte, H; Frenken, LGJ; Iturriza-gómara, M; Kiyono, H; Hammarström, L; Yuki, Y. "*Rice-based oral antibody fragment prophylaxis and therapy against rotavirus infection*," vol. 123, no. 9, 2013.

[6] Garaicoechea, L; Olichon, A; Marcoppido, G; Wigdorovitz, A; Mozgovoj, M; Saif, L; Surrey, T; Parreño, V. "Llama-derived single-chain antibody fragments directed to rotavirus VP6 protein possess broad neutralizing activity in vitro and confer protection against diarrhea in mice.," *J. Virol.*, vol. 82, no. 19, 9753–64, Oct. 2008.

[7] Aladin, F; Einerhand, AWC; Bouma, J; Bezemer, S; Hermans, P; Wolvers, D; Bellamy, K; Frenken, LGJ; Gray, J; Iturriza-Gómara, M. "In vitro neutralisation of rotavirus infection by two broadly specific recombinant monovalent llama-derived antibody fragments.," *PLoS One*, vol. 7, no. 3, p. e32949, Jan. 2012.

[8] Vega, CG; Bok, M; Vlasova, AN; Chattha, KS; Gómez-Sebastián, S; Nuñez, C; Alvarado, C; Lasa, R; Escribano, JM; Garaicoechea, LL; Fernandez, F; Bok, K; Wigdorovitz, A; Saif, LJ; Parreño, V. "Recombinant monovalent llama-derived antibody fragments (VHH) to rotavirus VP6 protect neonatal gnotobiotic piglets against human rotavirus-induced diarrhea.," *PLoS Pathog.*, vol. 9, no. 5, p. e1003334, Jan. 2013.

[9] Sarker, S; Jäkel, M; Sultana, S; Alam, NH; Bardhan, PK; Chisti, MJ; a Salam, M; Theis, W; Hammarström, L; Frenken, LGJ. "Anti-rotavirus protein reduces stool output in infants with diarrhea: a randomized placebo-controlled trial.," *Gastroenterology*, vol. 145, no. 4, 740–748.e8, Oct. 2013.

[10] Vanlandschoot, P; Stortelers, C; Beirnaert, E; Ibañez, LI; Schepens, B; Depla, E; Saelens, X. "Nanobodies®: new ammunition to battle viruses.," *Antiviral Res.*, vol. 92, no. 3, 389–407, Dec. 2011.

[11] Ewert, S; Cambillau, C; Conrath, K; Plückthun, A. "Biophysical properties of camelid VHH domains compared to those of human VH3 domains," *Biochemistry*, vol. 41, 3628–3636, 2002.

[12] Govaert, J; Pellis, M; Deschacht, N; Vincke, C; Conrath, K; Muyldermans, S; Saerens, D. "Dual Beneficial Effect of Interloop Disulfide Bond for Single Domain Antibody Fragments," *Journal of Biological Chemistry*, vol. 287. 1970–1979, 2012.

[13] Trilling, AK; Harmsen, MM; Ruigrok, VJB; Zuilhof, H; Beekwilder, J. "The effect of uniform capture molecule orientation on biosensor sensitivity: Dependence on analyte properties," *Biosens. Bioelectron.*, vol. 40, 219–226, 2013.

[14] Romer, T; Leonhardt, H; Rothbauer, U. "Engineering antibodies and proteins for molecular in vivo imaging," *Current Opinion in Biotechnology*, vol. 22. 882–887, 2011.

[15] Olichon, A. Surrey, T. "Selection of genetically encoded fluorescent single domain antibodies engineered for efficient expression in Escherichia coli.," *J. Biol. Chem.*, vol. 282, 36314–36320, 2007.

[16] Vaneycken, I; D' Huyvetter, M; Hernot, S; de Vos, J; Xavier, C; Devoogdt, N; Caveliers, V; Lahoutte, T. "Immuno-imaging using nanobodies," *Current Opinion in Biotechnology*, vol. 22. 877–881, 2011.

[17] Pauw. D. "Nanobodies and their potential applications P erspective," 1013–1026.

[18] van der Vaart, JM; Pant, N; Wolvers, D; Bezemer, S; Hermans, PW; Bellamy, K; a Sarker, S; van der Logt, CPE; Svensson, L; Verrips, CT; Hammarstrom, L; van Klinken, BJW. "Reduction in morbidity of rotavirus induced diarrhoea in mice by yeast produced monovalent llama-derived antibody fragments.," *Vaccine*, vol. 24, no. 19, 4130–7, May 2006.

[19] Matthijnssens, J; Otto, PH; Ciarlet, M; Desselberger, U; van Ranst, M; Johne, R. "VP6-sequence-based cutoff values as a criterion for rotavirus species demarcation," *Arch. Virol.*, vol. 157, 1177–1182, 2012.

[20] Tosser, G; Delaunay, T; Kohli, E; Grosclaude, J; Pothier, P; Cohen, J. "Topology of bovine rotavirus (RF strain) VP6 epitopes by real-time biospecific interaction analysis," *Virology*, vol. 204, no. 1, 8–16, 1994.

[21] Fleming, FE; Graham, KL; Taniguchi, K; Takada, Y; Coulson, BS. "Rotavirus-neutralizing antibodies inhibit virus binding to integrins alpha 2 beta 1 and alpha 4 beta 1," *Arch Virol*, vol. 152, no. 6, 1087–1101, 2007.

[22] Redmond, MJ; Ijaz, MK; Parker, MD; Sabara, MI; Dent, D; Gibbons, E; Babiuk, LA. "Assembly of recombinant rotavirus proteins into virus-like particles and assessment of vaccine potential," *Vaccine*, vol. 11, no. 2, 273–281, 1993.

[23] Feng, N; Lawton, JA; Gilbert, J; Kuklin, N; Vo, P; V Prasad, B; Greenberg, HB. "Inhibition of rotavirus replication by a non-neutralizing, rotavirus VP6-specific IgA mAb," *J Clin Invest*, vol. 109, no. 9, 1203–1213, 2002.

[24] Burns, JW; Siadat-Pajouh, M; Krishnaney, AA; Greenberg, HB. "Protective effect of rotavirus VP6-specific IgA monoclonal antibodies that lack neutralizing activity," *Science (80-.).*, vol. 272, no. 5258, 104–107, 1996.

[25] De Genst, E; Saerens, D; Muyldermans, S; Conrath, K. "Antibody repertoire development in camelids," *Dev. Comp. Immunol.*, vol. 30, 187–198, 2006.

[26] Estes, M. "Rotavirus and their replication (Cap 54a)," in *Fields Virology*, D. M. K. B. N. Fields P. M. Howley, Ed. Philadelphia: Lippincott - Raven, 2001.

[27] Gómez-Sebastián, S; Nuñez, MC; Garaicoechea, L; Alvarado, C; Mozgovoj, M; Lasa, R; Kahl, A; Wigdorovitz, A; Parreño, V; Escribano, JM. "Rotavirus A-specific single-domain antibodies produced in baculovirus-infected insect larvae are protective in vivo.," *BMC Biotechnol.*, vol. 12, p. 59, Jan. 2012.

[28] Lentz, EM; Garaicoechea, L; Alfano, EF; Parreño, V; Wigdorovitz, A; Bravo-Almonacid, FF. "Translational fusion and redirection to thylakoid lumen as strategies to improve the accumulation of a camelid antibody fragment in transplastomic tobacco.," *Planta*, vol. 236, no. 2, 703–14, Aug. 2012.

[29] Allen, SJ; Martinez, EG; Gregorio, GV; Dans, LF. "Probiotics for treating acute infectious diarrhoea.," *Cochrane Database Syst. Rev.*, p. CD003048, 2010.

[30] Krüger, C; Hultberg, A; van Dollenweerd, C; Marcotte, H; Hammarström, L. "Passive immunization by lactobacilli expressing single-chain antibodies against Streptococcus mutans.," *Mol. Biotechnol.*, vol. 31, 221–231, 2005.

[31] Pouwels, PH; Leer, RJ; Boersma, WJA. "The potential of Lactobacillus as a carrier for oral immunization: Development and preliminary characterization of vector systems for targeted delivery of antigens," in *Journal of Biotechnology*, 1996, vol. 44, 183–192.

[32] Hultberg, A; Zhao, Y; Svensson, L; Pan-Hammarstrom, Q; Johansen, K; Pouwels, PH; Ruggeri, FM; Hermans, P; Frenken, L; Boren, T; Marcotte, H; Hammarstrom, L. "Lactobacilli expressing variable domain of llama heavy-chain antibody fragments (lactobodies) confer protection against rotavirus-induced diarrhea.," *J. Infect. Dis.*, vol. 194, no. 11, 1580–8, Dec. 2006.

[33] Pant, N; Marcotte, H; Hermans, P; Bezemer, S; Frenken, L; Johansen, K. "Research Article," 583–593, 2011.

[34] Martín, MC; Pant, N; Ladero, V; Günaydin, G; Andersen, KK; Alvarez, B; Martínez, N; a Alvarez, M; Hammarström, L; Marcotte, H. "Integrative expression system for delivery of antibody fragments by lactobacilli.," *Appl. Environ. Microbiol.*, vol. 77, no. 6, 2174–9, Mar. 2011.

[35] Burns, JW; Krishnaney, AA; Vo, PT; Rouse, RV; Anderson, LJ; Greenberg, HB. "Analyses of homologous rotavirus infection in the mouse model.," *Virology*, vol. 207, 143–153, 1995.

[36] Saif, LJ; Ward, LA; Yuan, L; Rosen, BI; To, TL. "The gnotobiotic piglet as a model for studies of disease pathogenesis and immunity to human rotaviruses," *Arch Virol Suppl*, vol. 12, 153–161, 1996.

[37] Franco, MA; Angel, J; Greenberg, HB. "Immunity and correlates of protection for rotavirus vaccines," *Vaccine*, vol. 24, no. 15, 2718–2731, 2006.

[38] Yuan, L; Saif, LJ. "Induction of mucosal immune responses and protection against enteric viruses: Rotavirus infection of gnotobiotic pigs as a model," in *Veterinary Immunology and Immunopathology*, 2002, vol. 87, 147–160.

In: Rotavirus Infections
Editor: Carissa D. Zeni
ISBN: 978-1-63321-442-2

Chapter 7

Neurological Presentation of Rotavirus Infection: Epidemiology and Possible Pathophysiology

Jung Sook Yeom and Hee-Shang Youn
Department of Pediatrics,
Gyeongsang National University School of Medicine,
Gyeongsang Institute of Health Science, Jinju, Korea

Abstract

Rotavirus infections are the most common cause of infant and childhood gastroenteritis. However, a number of neurological manifestations, ranging from benign seizures to lethal encephalitis, have been observed during the course of the infection. Afebrile seizures following gastroenteritis are the most common neurological symptom of rotavirus infection, occurring in 2.1–6.4% of patients with rotavirus gastroenteritis. Furthermore, rotavirus may be a causative pathogen associated with a spectrum of encephalitis disorders including clinically mild encephalitis/encephalopathy with a reversible splenial lesion, cerebellitis, and acute necrotizing encephalopathy. Furthermore, rotavirus may play a role in neonatal seizures, particularly in relation to the 'fifth day fit'. The epidemiology and clinical manifestations of rotavirus gastroenteritis-associated seizures changed after introduction of the rotavirus vaccine. This chapter reviews the neurological presentation and epidemiology of the rotavirus infection with a focus on rotavirus-associated seizures, potential pathogenic mechanisms, treatment, and prognosis. We discuss the impact of the rotavirus vaccine on childhood seizures and possible underlying mechanisms.

1. Introduction

Rotavirus infections are the most common cause of infant and childhood gastroenteritis. Rotavirus-associated gastroenteritis may be accompanied by a spectrum of neurological manifestations ranging from benign febrile/afebrile seizures to lethal encephalopathy/encephalitis. [1,2] These symptoms are relatively common, occurring in approximately 1.7–6.4% of patients.[3,4,5] However, the way in which rotavirus spreads to the central nerve system (CNS) and the long-term prognosis of rotavirus-associated neurological manifestations are not known. This chapter reviews the neurological presentation and epidemiology of the rotavirus infection with a focus on rotavirus-associated seizures, potential pathogenic mechanisms, treatment, and prognosis. We discuss the impact of the rotavirus vaccine on childhood seizures and possible underlying mechanisms.

2. Epidemiology

Benign seizures are the most common neurological symptom associated with rotavirus infection. Several large observational studies have reported the prevalence of benign febrile/afebrile seizures following rotavirus gastroenteritis to be between 4.0 and 7.7%. [3, 6, 7] The incidence of rotavirus-associated seizures differs depending upon whether the infection is accompanied by fever. Lloyd et al. [6] found that the overall prevalence of seizures among hospitalized children was 4.6 per 100 rotavirus-infected children; however, the prevalence of febrile seizures was 0.9% (12 children with febrile seizures among 1,292 with a rotavirus infection). Similarly, Kang et al. [7] found the prevalence of febrile and afebrile seizures associated with rotavirus to be 2.2 and 5.5%, respectively. Thus, rotavirus-associated afebrile seizures appear to be more prevalent than febrile seizures.

Few studies have investigated the incidence/prevalence of rotavirus-associated encephalopathy/encephalitis, and the incidence of the condition is not known. A large Swedish surveillance study [3] found a 1.7% prevalence of encephalitis with abnormal electroencephalogram (EEG) results in 984 children hospitalized with rotavirus gastroenteritis over an 11-year period. The estimated annual rate of rotavirus-associated encephalopathy/encephalitis cases in Japan is 44 per year. [8] A nationwide Japanese survey [9] conducted by Hoshino et al. revealed that rotavirus was the third most common pathogen associated with acute encephalopathy/encephalitis in Japanese children. Furthermore, rotavirus was the pathogenic virus in 18 of 983 cases (1.8%) of encephalopathy. Of the 18 cases of rotavirus-associated encephalopathy/ encephalitis, clinically mild encephalitis/encephalopathy with a reversible splenial lesion was most common (45.0%), followed by acute encephalopathy with biphasic seizures and later reduced diffusion (10.0%), and acute necrotizing encephalopathy of childhood (2.5%). [9] Rotavirus cerebellitis is included in the spectrum of rotavirus infections; however, the incidence has not been investigated.

3. Rotavirus-Associated Seizures with Afebrile Benign Convulsion with Mild Gastroenteritis (CWG): A Distinct Clinical Entity

3.1. Clinical Features

An association between afebrile seizures and diarrheal illness has been suspected for several decades. [10-13] Japanese neuropediatricians now recognize afebrile convulsions triggered by mild diarrhea in infants and young children as a distinct clinical entity referred to as convulsion with mild gastroenteritis (CwG). [14] CwG is characterized by convulsions accompanying mild diarrhea without dehydration or electrolyte derangement, and fever before and after the seizures, in previously healthy infants and children with no evidence of CNS infection. [10, 14] Although CwG can be caused by various infectious pathogens, rotavirus is the primary cause of the condition. Rotavirus has been detected in 54–70% of stool samples in CwG cases, [15-16] and the relative risk of seizure with diarrhea is highest when rotavirus is detected in stool specimens. [17] The relative risk of patients with rotavirus gastroenteritis developing a seizure has been reported to be 2.3 compared with a negative culture and 1.8 compared with bacteria enteritis.

[17] We will review the overall clinical features of CwG, and then discuss studies comparing afebrile and febrile seizures in patients with a rotavirus infection.

CwG occurs in previously healthy and normally developed infants and young children between 6 months and 4 years of age. [10] The condition commonly occurs in children 1 to 2 years of age, [18] and the mean age of patients affected by rotavirus-associated CwG is 17–22 months. [6, 7, 18, 19] The gastroenteritis symptoms are generally mild, and most children show no clinical evidence of more than 5% dehydration. [10, 16] No association has been found between the duration or severity of diarrhea and the number or duration of seizures. The mean interval between the onset of gastroenteritis and seizures has been reported to be 2.4–2.8 days. [7, 19] Seizures most often occur 3 days after the onset of diarrhea and rarely occur later than day 4. [14, 16, 18] However, a seizure may occur before the onset of diarrhea. [20]

Generalized tonic-clonic seizures (GTC) are the most common seizure type associated with CwG and rotavirus-related CwG. [7, 14, 15, 18, 21] However, several lines of evidence suggest that GTC seizures in patients with CwG may be the result of secondarily generalized partial seizures. [21, 22] Seizures with focal features similar to those of complex partial seizures, such as lateral eye deviation and hemiconvulsion, have been observed in patients with CwG. [7, 10, 15, 23] Cusmai et al., [24] found that direct observation of seizure semiology in patients with CwG indicated partial seizures with secondary generalization, whereas the description given by the parents suggested generalized seizures. Moreover, the fact that few ictal EEGs have been reported in patients with CwG supports the theory that GTCs are the result of partial seizures with secondary generalization, primarily originating in the centro-parieto-occipital regions [24-26]. CwG seizures are brief (<5 min in 85% of cases); [14, 18] however, they characteristically occur in clusters ranging from one to eight episodes in a 24-h period. [7, 14, 18] Two or more seizures develop in 67.5–85.7% of patients with CwG. [7, 18]. The characteristic clustering afebrile partial seizures should alert clinicians to the diagnosis of CwG, particularly when the seizures occur prior to the onset of diarrhea.

Although rotavirus gastroenteritis is associated with fever, and febrile seizures may occur during the illness, most case series have focused on afebrile seizures. A few studies have investigated the clinical distinctions between febrile and afebrile seizures associated with rotavirus gastroenteritis. [6, 7] Lloyd et al., [6] found no difference in median age, sex, race distribution, or median length of hospital stay between febrile and afebrile seizure groups. Additionally, these authors found no between-group differences in duration and type of seizures. However, Kang et al., [7] reported that the duration of gastrointestinal symptoms before the onset of seizures was significantly longer, seizure frequency was significantly higher, and focal features were significantly more prevalent in patients who experienced febrile seizures than in those with afebrile seizures. Their findings indicate that the presence of fever can affect the seizure characteristics and suggest that rotavirus-associated febrile and afebrile seizures are distinct clinical entities. Further prospective studies with large sample are necessary to confirm the effect of fever on rotavirus-related seizures.

3.2. Investigations

The few studies that have investigated laboratory, radiological, and EEG findings in patients rotavirus gastroenteritis-associated seizures, [7, 18, 19, 27, 28] reported that most laboratory results, including cerebral spinal fluid (CSF), were within the normal range. However, several authors have noted that the laboratory features of patients with rotavirus-associated CwG differed from those of patients who had febrile seizures or rotavirus gastroenteritis with no seizures. Motoyama et al. [27] reported that serum Na^+ and Cl^- were significantly lower in patients with rotavirus-associated CwG than in those with a seizure-free rotavirus infection, although the Na^+ and Cl^- levels were within the normal range. Based on these findings, Motoyama et al., [28] hypothesized that rotavirus-associated CwG involved Na+ channels, which explains why carbamazepine is an effective therapy for CwG. In a previous study, we compared the laboratory results of rotavirus gastroenteritis patients with and without seizures. [19] We found that serum Na^+ and Cl^- levels were lower in patients without seizures than in those who had seizures; however, the difference was not statistically significant. Alternatively, we found that serum Ca^{2+} levels were significantly lower in the patients with than in those without seizures. Thus, we proposed that disruption of Ca^{2+} homeostasis may play a role in the development of seizures in patients with rotavirus gastroenteritis. We will discuss this hypothesis in the pathophysiology section of our chapter. Nevertheless, it is clear that relatively low Na^+ and Ca^{2+} levels alone do not directly cause rotavirus-associated seizures.

Ictal EEGs have revealed focal onset seizures evolving to secondary generalization. [24-26]. The onset of ictal discharge was most frequently observed in the posterior cerebral areas. [24-26] In a recent study, Cusmai et al.[24] performed ictal EEG recordings in four children. The seizures showed focal onset in the left central region in one patient, in the right parieto-occipital region in two patients, and in the left occipital region in one patient. Occipital, parietal, and central areas are hyper excitable brain regions that may be involved in an age-related, benign childhood seizure susceptibility syndrome. Cusmai and colleagues concluded that, similar to other benign focal infantile convulsions, CwG seizures can be partial and involve different brain areas. Imai et al., [25] studied ictal-video EEG recordings of a cluster of three seizures in a 6-month-old infant. They found that all seizures began as complex partial seizures, which exhibited a motionless stare with or without leftward deviation of both eyes, and evolved to secondarily generalized GTC seizures. Interestingly, each of the three ictal discharges began in different brain regions, from the right occipital, right centro-parieto-temporal, and left occipital regions. These findings are consistent with those of Cusmai et al., [24] and support the hypothesis that CwG seizures are initiated in hyper excitable brain regions involved in an age-related, benign childhood seizure susceptibility syndrome.

To summarize, the bulk of the evidence indicates that CwG-related seizures arise from focal regions in posterior brain areas. However, the inter-ictal EEG was found to be normal in most cases, [6, 7, 19, 23, 24] including those showing focal epileptiform activity, which was normalized in follow-up EEGs. [7, 18]

Although neuroimaging is not required for the diagnosis of CwG, those with rotavirus-associated seizures and no fever are more likely to undergo neuroimaging than children with seizures and fever. [6] The repetitive afebrile seizures characteristic of CwG may cause concern, prompting clinicians to use neuroimaging, typically computed tomography, to assess those patients. [10, 15, 16, 26] However, magnetic resonance imaging (MRI) may detect a transient splenial lesion of the corpus callosum [7,19]. Given that rotavirus is one of the most common causes of clinically mild encephalitis/encephalopathy with a reversible splenial lesion, the decision to use MRI to diagnosis CwG is reasonable [9].

The diagnosis of CwG is based on clinical findings; thus, laboratory investigations may appear to be unnecessary. However, Difazio et al., [29] recommended that patients with CwG undergo standard testing for a first-time seizure, given the co-occurrence of rotavirus, which is a fairly common viral illness. They suggested that a child who presented with ongoing or clusters of seizures in association with rotavirus gastroenteritis should be admitted to hospital for stabilization and diagnostic testing. Furthermore, the authors recommended EEG and electrolyte screening under these circumstances. Verrotti et al., [14] recommended lumbar puncture, serum electrolyte analysis, and serial EEGs for selected cases, such as patients with a cluster of seizures. We maintain that CwG should be diagnosed only after the clinical and laboratory criteria for CwG are met.

3.3. Pathophysiology

The cause of rotavirus-associated seizures is not known. Several mechanisms may underlie the neurological symptoms in children with rotavirus gastroenteritis, such as 1) the rotavirus itself, directly or secondarily, 2) abnormal electrolyte imbalance or dehydration, 3) fever, and 4) a spectrum of age-related, benign childhood seizure susceptibility syndrome. Patients with rotavirus-associated seizures typically do not have serious electrolyte or metabolic imbalances and they are generally afebrile. [29] Thus, the most likely cause of the seizures associated with the rotavirus infection is CNS involvement in children who have a genetic susceptibility to seizures. First we review evidence for CNS involvement, and then we discuss the possibility of genetic susceptibility and an age-related, benign childhood seizure susceptibility syndrome as a cause of rotavirus-associated seizures.

The hypothesis that rotavirus-associated seizures are caused by direct CNS invasion by the virus is supported by the detection of rotavirus in the CSF using reverse transcriptase-PCR or enzyme-linked immunosorbent assay (ELISA). [30, 31] However, it is necessary to determine how the virus enters the bloodstream, crosses the blood-brain-barrier, and causes seizures to confirm the hypothesis. Several studies have detected rotavirus RNA or antigen in the blood. [32, 33] Antigenemia and viremia have been detected in 45–50 [34, 35] and 5% [34] of patients with rotavirus gastroenteritis, respectively. Exanthema detected in 4% of infected patients may provide further evidence of viremia in rotavirus gastroenteritis. [36] These findings suggest that rotavirus can escape the intestinal tract in children resulting in antigenemia and possible viremia. Seizures are related to the peak viral load in stool, [19] and the level of viremia is directly associated with antigen levels in stool [37]. Although viremia may explain the extraintestinal manifestations of rotavirus infection, particularly seizures, the question of how the rotavirus enters the bloodstream remains. The detection of rotavirus-specific proteins in macrophages and B cells in gut-associated lymphoid tissue after oral inoculation suggests that the virus may travel to distant sites via lymphoid tissue in gut [38]. However, disagreement exists as to whether antigenemia and viremia are associated with extraintestinal manifestations of the rotavirus. Several studies have found that children with antigenemia had more severe symptoms or higher fever than children without antigenemia, but not a higher incidence of extraintestinal presentations [32, 35]. Moreover, most rotavirus gastroenteritis-associated seizures are afebrile and accompanied by mild symptoms of gastroenteritis, which is not consistent with the clinical features of antigenemia or viremia. Finally, a systemic inflammatory reaction has not been reported in rotavirus gastroenteritis-associated seizures [19]. Thus, the presence of antigenemia or viremia alone does not provide direct evidence for the extraintestinal manifestation of rotavirus infection. Further studies are necessary to clarify this issue.

It is not known how rotavirus crosses the brain-blood-barrier, and it may be that the rotavirus detected in the CSF is the result of seizures rather than their cause. Increased blood-brain-barrier permeability during seizures may allow the virus to enter the CSF. [39]. We believe that an interaction between brain mast cells and the enteric nervous system plays an important role in rotavirus gastroenteritis-associated seizures. Rotavirus infection triggers the release of neurotransmitters such as neurotensin [40]. Neurotensin stimulates mast cells to release vasodilatory and inflammatory mediators (including interlukin-6), some of which increase the expression of vascular endothelial cell adhesion molecules and permit circulating virus-laden lymphocytes to enter the brain. [41]. Moreover, neurotensin can facilitate N-Methyl-D-aspartate (NMDA)-induced excitation of cortical neurons [42] and seizure activity in rodents [43]. Thus, the brain-gut axis may provide the answer to how rotavirus crosses the brain-blood-barrier and causes seizures in the brain. Furthermore, our brain-gut interaction hypothesis can explain why pleocytosis is not evident in the CSF of most rotavirus-associated seizure cases, and the increase in CSF IL-6 in the absence of rotavirus. Thus, the hypothesis explains an indirect effect of rotavirus in the CNS. However, several studies have shown that the virus can directly affect the CNS. Rotavirus has been shown to infect neurons *in vitro* [44] and *in vivo* [45]. Direct inoculation of rotavirus is associated with neurological compromise and histological evidence of infection. [46] However, this evidence is not sufficient to prove that rotavirus itself induces seizures.

Finally, an indirect or secondary effect of the virus in the brain may explain how rotavirus causes seizures. A rotavirus enterotoxin may play a key role as a neurotoxic mediator. Rotavirus infection modifies Ca^{2+} homeostasis, which plays a critical role in the induction of enterocyte cell death and causes diarrhea through a multifactorial process involving Ca^{2+}-dependent secretory mediators, water, and electrolytes. [47] A progressive increase in the permeability of plasma membrane Ca^{2+} leads to an elevation in cytoplasmic Ca^{2+} concentration and an increase in sequestered Ca^{2+} pools in the endoplasmic reticulum [48]. The non-structural protein, NSP4, may be responsible for these effects. NSP4-mediated Ca^{2+} mobilization triggers the release of amines, peptides, cytokines, prostaglandins, nitric oxide, and reactive oxygen species [29]. These mediators may induce diarrhea as well as seizures. Nitric oxide is markedly elevated in the CSF of patients with rotavirus-associated seizures, [49] and an excessive amount of the molecule in the CNS can induce limbic seizures and delayed hippocampal neuronal damage [49]. Rotavirus infection stimulates nitric oxide production during the course of the disease [50]. NSP4 can stimulate inducible nitric oxide synthase expression in the intestine and macrophages [51]. A recent study revealed that NSP4 stimulates the release of serotonin from human enterochromaffin cells and activates brain structures involved in nausea and vomiting [52]. These findings suggest that CNS-affecting mediators can be synthesized by NSP4 action in the intestine, which may trigger rotavirus-associated seizures. In a previous study, we found that Ca^{2+} levels were significantly lower in patients with rotavirus-associated seizures than in those without seizures [19].

We hypothesized that disruption of Ca^{2+} homeostasis can be gaged by serum Ca^{2+} levels. It is not clear whether an influx of Ca^{2+} caused by an increase in plasma membrane permeability can decrease serum levels of Ca^{2+}; however, our assumption may hold true if Ca^{2+} influx occurs in a sufficient number of enterocytes. Low serum Cl^- levels observed in patients who had seizures may further support our hypothesis because an increase in intracellular Ca^{2+} is involved in the induction of diarrhea via a Ca^{2+}-dependent Cl^- secretory mechanism. Although Ca^{2+} levels were within the normal range and did not directly cause seizures in our study, we postulated a role for NSP4 in rotavirus-associated seizures based on the association between the disruption of Ca^{2+} homeostasis and seizures in patients with rotavirus [19]. Alternatively, NSP4 itself may be released from infected enterocytes via secretion or lysis [47]. A high prevalence of NSP4 genes in acute-phase peripheral blood mononuclear cells was reported recently [53]. Moreover, NSP4 has been found to be widely distributed in neuronal cell bodies and dendrites [44]. These findings suggest that rotavirus may replicate in white blood cells, thus, allowing the extraintestinal spread of NSP4. Given the membrane-destabilizing properties of NSP4, a direct effect of the protein in the CNS is plausible. However, no evidence exists for a role of NSP4 in rotavirus-associated seizures. Furthermore, it is not clear how distinctive anatomical locations (i.e., brain vs. gut) are linked to events in enterocytes. Nevertheless, we believe that the NSP4 protein is the most likely mediator of rotavirus-associated seizures based on its properties (i.e., neurotransmitter dysregulation, membrane-destabilizing activity, and increased intracellular Ca^{2+} levels). [54, 55]. We believe this hypothesis warrants further investigation.

Few studies have clearly demonstrated a familial or genetic predisposition to CwG. [24, 56] Sakai et al., [56] described CwG in siblings whose father and grandfather had infantile convulsions, suggesting a genetically determined susceptibility to seizures during mild gastroenteritis. Although a specific genetic trait has not been identified, rotavirus-associated seizures and CwG are similar to other benign epileptic childhood syndromes. [24]. The dramatic appearance of clusters of focal seizures, often lasting several days, in previously healthy children is a common feature of other benign childhood epileptic syndromes [24]. Moreover, the characteristics of rotavirus-associated seizures and CwG overlap considerably with those of febrile convulsions, such as occurring only at a young age (6 months to 4 years), rare seizure recurrence, normal development, and no future epilepsy. Although the pathogenesis of febrile seizures is multifactorial, several studies have demonstrated a genetic predisposition. Linkage studies have identified 11 chromosomal locations responsible for febrile seizures [57]. The SCN1A, IL-1β, CHRNA4, and GABRG2 genes are most frequently involved in febrile seizures [57]. These findings suggest that rotavirus-associated seizures and CwG have a genetic predisposition or are linked with an age-related, benign childhood seizure susceptibility syndrome. In summary, rotavirus may induce seizure via direct or indirect action in the CNS in genetically susceptible children.

3.4. Treatment

Anticonvulsant therapy is not necessary for patients who experience a single seizure because such seizures are generally brief. However, rotavirus-associated seizures and CwG frequently occur in clusters and are refractory to antiepileptic drugs.

Diazepam is widely used as the first-line treatment for convulsive conditions because it acts rapidly. However, Okamura et al., [58] reported that diazepam failed to stop seizures in the majority of patients with CwG. In their study, diazepam was administered as the first-treatment for all patients;

however, the drug was effective in only 39 patients. Omata et al., [59] found that seizures recurred in 65% of patients treated with diazepam. Similarly, Hayashi et al., [60] reported that diazepam was effective in two of nine patients with CwG who had a clusters of seizures. Thus, diazepam is not recommended for the treatment of CwG [14].

Phenobarbital is used as the first- or second-line treatment for convulsions. In contrast to diazepam, phenobarbital is relatively effective in patients with CwG. [58] Omata et al., [59] reported that 10–15 mg/kg of phenobarbital was effective for the prevention of clustering seizures in all patients with CwG. Although a large dose of phenobarbital may be effective, the adverse effects of the drug may increase [58].

Carbamazepine can control CwG. Ichiyama et al., [61] found that low-dose carbamazepine (5 mg/kg/day) was effective in 15 of 16 cases (93.7%). Motoyama et al., [27] reported that low-dose carbamazepine was effective in 12 of 13 patients with CwG. They found that serum Na^+ and Cl^- levels were lower in patients with CwG than in those without seizures. The authors concluded that carbamazepine was effective for patients with CwG because it blocked Na^+ channels. Like carbamazepine, lidocaine is a Na^+ channel blocker. Okumura et al., [58] reported that lidocaine was 100% effective in controlling seizures in patents with CwG and significantly more effective than diazepam and phenobarbital; however, their sample size was small. These findings suggest that antiepileptic drugs that block Na^+ channels are an effective treatment for CwG. However, large, prospective, randomized, case-control studies are needed to identify the optimal antiepileptic drug for stopping seizures in CwG. [14] In summary, treatment with antiepileptic drugs is indicated to stop cluster seizures; however, the medication is unlikely to influence the long-term prognosis of the patients. Thus, chronic treatment with antiepileptic drugs should be avoided in patients with CwG.

3.5. Impact of the Rotavirus Vaccine

Uptake of the rotavirus vaccine into the national immunization program of several countries has resulted in a sustained reduction in the prevalence of rotavirus infection and diarrhea-related mortality and/or morbidity. [62] Moreover, changes have been observed in the circulating virus strains and the timing of the rotavirus season since introduction of the rotavirus vaccine [63]. The rotavirus season appears to be delayed, shorter, and diminished in magnitude [64]. Furthermore, the epidemiological impact of the rotavirus vaccine has been observed in regions with low and moderate vaccine uptake, such as Germany and Korea [65, 66]. It is possible that the epidemiological impact of the vaccine has influenced the clinical features of rotavirus gastroenteritis-associated seizures. Thus, we investigated whether the clinical features of rotavirus-associated seizures changed following introduction of rotavirus vaccine in Korea. Our study included pediatric patients between 6 months and 5 years of age who presented with seizures during the course of rotavirus-associated gastroenteritis. The patients were divided into two groups according to the introduction of the rotavirus in Korea: pre-vaccine period (July 2002 to June 2006) and the post-vaccine period (July 2008 to June 2013). We compared clinical data of the groups (age, sex, season of hospital visit, body temperature just before or after seizures, interval between onset of gastroenteritis symptoms and onset of seizures, previous history of seizure, and family history of febrile seizure and epilepsy). We found that the seizure characteristics were significantly different between groups: the post-vaccine group had a lower incidence of fever at the time of seizure, a longer interval between the development of gastroenteritis symptoms and seizure onset, and higher frequency of seizures than the pre-vaccine group [67]. These characteristics suggest that seizure susceptibility was increased in the post-vaccine period. However, we detected no significant between-group differences in age, sex, previous febrile convulsion history, or family history of febrile convulsion and epilepsy, suggesting that the changes were not the result of individual differences in genetic seizure susceptibility. Only one patient in our study was inoculated with the rotavirus vaccine; thus, the changes in seizure characteristics were not related to the direct effects of the vaccine. We excluded patients under the age of 6 months from the study to minimize the role of maternal antibodies to rotavirus; thus, maternal antibodies should not have affected the observed changes in the clinical characteristics of the rotavirus-associated seizures. Further studies are needed to determine the cause of the changes in rotavirus-associated seizures following the introduction of the rotavirus vaccine in Korea. In our study, 70% (31 of 44) of patients with rotavirus gastroenteritis in the pre-vaccine group experienced seizures compared with 9.7% (25 of 257) of patients in the post-vaccine group [67]. Although the proportion of seizures was significantly greater in the post- than the pre-vaccine group, the absolute number of patients with seizures was only slightly reduced after introduction of the rotavirus vaccine. Our findings are consistent with a recent epidemiological study conducted by Payne et al., [68] in the United States. The authors reported that a full course of rotavirus vaccine was associated with a significant (18–21%) reduction in the risk of seizures requiring hospitalization or emergency department care in the year following vaccination. Weinberg [69] noted that the magnitude of the effect of rotavirus vaccination on early childhood seizures reported by Payne and colleagues was surprisingly large considering that ≤7% of medically attended children with rotavirus gastroenteritis have been reported to have a seizure. However, Weinberg suggested that the "extra protection" of the 20% reduction in seizure incidence reported by Payne et al. could be explained by the likelihood that the proportion of seizures thought to be associated with rotavirus has been underestimated, and suggested that results of Payne et al. lent further support to the call for universal rotavirus immunization. However, the indirect effects of the rotavirus vaccine on seizures, and the increased susceptibility to seizure in unvaccinated children, as we have shown in unpublished data, warrants further evaluation.

3.6. Prognosis

Rotavirus-associated seizures are generally benign. Although most studies have not followed patients beyond 2.5–3 years, follow-up EEG and psychomotor development have been reported to be normal. [10, 15, 16] According to Lee and Ong, [12] who recorded the longest follow-up period, the Kaplan-Meier estimate of risk at 5 years for subsequent unprovoked afebrile seizures after a first febrile, provoked, or unprovoked afebrile seizures was 0.9%, 6.2%, and 62.3% respectively. Thus, patients in whom gastroenteritis was the cause of provoked afebrile seizures had a significantly lower risk of subsequent unprovoked seizures than did patients who had a respiratory infection or nonspecific febrile illness. The Kaplan-Meier estimate of risk at 5-year follow-up was 0.9% for gastroenteritis, 13.8% for respiratory infection, 19.0% for nonspecific febrile illness, and 2.4% for other infectious syndrome. These findings suggest that the CwG prognosis is similar to that of febrile seizures and that multiple seizures during the provoking illness, focality, and seizure duration are not associated with an adverse prognosis.

References

[1] Shiihara T, Watanabe M, Honma A, Kato M, Morita Y, Ichiyama T, et al. Rotavirus associated acute encephalitis/encephalopathy and

concurrent cerebellitis: Report of two cases. *Brain Dev.* 2007 Nov;29(10):670-3.

[2] Thompson MJ, Gowdie PJ, Kirkwood CD, Doherty RR, Fahey M. Rotavirus cerebellitis: New aspects to an old foe? *Pediatr. Neurol.* 2012 Jan;46(1):48-50.

[3] Johansen K, Hedlund KO, Zweygberg-Wirgart B, Bennet R. Complications attributable to rotavirus-induced diarrhoea in a swedish paediatric population: Report from an 11-year surveillance. *Scand. J. Infect Dis.* 2008;40(11-12):958-64.

[4] Huang CC, Chang YC, Wang ST. Acute symptomatic seizure disorders in young children--a population study in southern taiwan. *Epilepsia.* 1998 Sep;39(9):960-4.

[5] Iyadurai S, Troester M, Harmala J, Bodensteiner J. Benign afebrile seizures in acute gastroenteritis: Is rotavirus the culprit? *J. Child Neurol.* 2007 Jul;22(7):887-90.

[6] Lloyd MB, Lloyd JC, Gesteland PH, Bale JF,Jr. Rotavirus gastroenteritis and seizures in young children. *Pediatr. Neurol.* 2010 Jun;42(6):404-8.

[7] Kang B, Kim DH, Hong YJ, Son BK, Kim DW, Kwon YS. Comparison between febrile and afebrile seizures associated with mild rotavirus gastroenteritis. *Seizure.* 2013 Sep;22(7):560-4.

[8] Kawamura Y, Ohashi M, Ihira M, Hashimoto S, Taniguchi K, Yoshikawa T. Nationwide survey of rotavirus-associated encephalopathy and sudden unexpected death in japan. *Brain Dev.* 2013 Aug 21.

[9] Hoshino A, Saitoh M, Oka A, Okumura A, Kubota M, Saito Y, et al. Epidemiology of acute encephalopathy in japan, with emphasis on the association of viruses and syndromes. *Brain Dev.* 2012 May;34(5):337-43.

[10] Komori H, Wada M, Eto M, Oki H, Aida K, Fujimoto T. Benign convulsions with mild gastroenteritis: A report of 10 recent cases detailing clinical varieties. *Brain Dev.* 1995 Sep-Oct;17(5):334-7.

[11] Fukuyama Y. Borderland of epilepsy with special reference to febrile convulsions and so-called infantile convulsions. *Seishin Igaku.* 1963;5:211-3.

[12] Lee WL, Ong HT. Afebrile seizures associated with minor infections: Comparison with febrile seizures and unprovoked seizures. *Pediatr Neurol.* 2004 Sep;31(3):157-64.

[13] Zerr DM, Blume HK, Berg AT, Del Beccaro MA, Gospe SM,Jr, Allpress AL, et al. Nonfebrile illness seizures: A unique seizure category? *Epilepsia*. 2005 Jun;46(6):952-5.
[14] Verrotti A, Tocco AM, Coppola GG, Altobelli E, Chiarelli F. Afebrile benign convulsions with mild gastroenteritis: A new entity? *Acta Neurol Scand*. 2009 Aug;120(2):73-9.
[15] Uemura N, Okumura A, Negoro T, Watanabe K. Clinical features of benign convulsions with mild gastroenteritis. *Brain Dev*. 2002 Dec;24(8):745-9.
[16] Narchi H. Benign afebrile cluster convulsions with gastroenteritis: An observational study. *BMC Pediatr*. 2004 Feb 5;4:2.
[17] Wong V. Acute gastroenteritis-related encephalopathy. *J. Child Neurol.* 2001 Dec;16(12):906-10.
[18] Hung JJ, Wen HY, Yen MH, Chen HW, Yan DC, Lin KL, et al. Rotavirus gastroenteritis associated with afebrile convulsion in children: Clinical analysis of 40 cases. *Chang Gung Med J*. 2003 Sep;26(9):654-9.
[19] Yeom JS, Kim YS, Park JS, Seo JH, Park ES, Lim JY, et al. Role of Ca2+ homeostasis disruption in rotavirus-associated seizures. *J. Child Neurol.* 2012 Dec 26.
[20] Dura-Trave T, Yoldi-Petri ME, Gallinas-Victoriano F, Molins-Castiella T. Infantile convulsions with mild gastroenteritis: A retrospective study of 25 patients. *Eur. J. Neurol*. 2011 Feb;18(2):273-8.
[21] Narchi H. Benign afebrile cluster convulsions with gastroenteritis: An observational study. *BMC Pediatr*. 2004 Feb 5;4:2.
[22] Abe T, Kobayashi M, Araki K, Kodama H, Fujita Y, Shinozaki T, et al. Infantile convulsions with mild gastroenteritis. *Brain Dev*. 2000 Aug;22(5):301-6.
[23] Caraballo RH, Ganez L, Santos Cde L, Espeche A, Cersosimo R, Fejerman N. Benign infantile seizures with mild gastroenteritis: Study of 22 patients. *Seizure*. 2009 Dec;18(10):686-9.
[24] Cusmai R, Jocic-Jakubi B, Cantonetti L, Japaridze N, Vigevano F. Convulsions associated with gastroenteritis in the spectrum of benign focal epilepsies in infancy: 30 cases including four cases with ictal EEG recording. *Epileptic Disord*. 2010 Dec;12(4):255-61.
[25] Imai K, Otani K, Yanagihara K, Li Z, Futagi Y, Ono J, et al. Ictal video-EEG recording of three partial seizures in a patient with the benign infantile convulsions associated with mild gastroenteritis. *Epilepsia.* 1999 Oct;40(10):1455-8.

[26] Maruyama K, Okumura A, Sofue A, Ishihara N, Watanabe K. Ictal EEG in patients with convulsions with mild gastroenteritis. *Brain Dev.* 2007 Jan;29(1):43-6.

[27] Motoyama M, Ichiyama T, Matsushige T, Kajimoto M, Shiraishi M, Furukawa S. Clinical characteristics of benign convulsions with rotavirus gastroenteritis. *J. Child Neurol.* 2009 May;24(5):557-61.

[28] Kawano G, Oshige K, Syutou S, Koteda Y, Yokoyama T, Kim BG, et al. Benign infantile convulsions associated with mild gastroenteritis: A retrospective study of 39 cases including virological tests and efficacy of anticonvulsants. *Brain Dev.* 2007 Nov;29(10):617-22.

[29] DiFazio MP, Braun L, Freedman S, Hickey P. Rotavirus-induced seizures in childhood. *J. Child Neurol.* 2007 Dec;22(12):1367-70.

[30] Nishimura S, Ushijima H, Nishimura S, Shiraishi H, Kanazawa C, Abe T, et al. Detection of rotavirus in cerebrospinal fluid and blood of patients with convulsions and gastroenteritis by means of the reverse transcription polymerase chain reaction. *Brain Dev.* 1993 Nov-Dec;15(6):457-9.

[31] Lynch M, Lee B, Azimi P, Gentsch J, Glaser C, Gilliam S, et al. Rotavirus and central nervous system symptoms: Cause or contaminant? case reports and review. *Clin. Infect Dis.* 2001 Oct 1;33(7):932-8.

[32] Sugata K, Taniguchi K, Yui A, Miyake F, Suga S, Asano Y, et al. Analysis of rotavirus antigenemia and extraintestinal manifestations in children with rotavirus gastroenteritis. *Pediatrics.* 2008 Aug;122(2):392-7.

[33] Liu B, Fujita Y, Arakawa C, Kohira R, Fuchigami T, Mugishima H, et al. Detection of rotavirus RNA and antigens in serum and cerebrospinal fluid samples from diarrheic children with seizures. *Jpn J. Infect Dis.* 2009 Jul;62(4):279-83.

[34] Yu TH, Tsai CN, Lai MW, Chen CC, Chao HC, Lin CW, et al. Antigenemia and cytokine expression in rotavirus gastroenteritis in children. *J. Microbiol Immunol Infect.* 2012 Aug;45(4):265-70.

[35] Ramani S, Sowmyanarayanan TV, Gladstone BP, Bhowmick K, Asirvatham JR, Jana AK, et al. Rotavirus infection in the neonatal nurseries of a tertiary care hospital in india. *Pediatr. Infect Dis J.* 2008 Aug;27(8):719-23.

[36] Gilger MA, Matson DO, Conner ME, Rosenblatt HM, Finegold MJ, Estes MK. Extraintestinal rotavirus infections in children with immunodeficiency. *J. Pediatr.* 1992 Jun;120(6):912-7.

[37] Blutt SE, Kirkwood CD, Parreno V, Warfield KL, Ciarlet M, Estes MK, et al. Rotavirus antigenaemia and viraemia: A common event? *Lancet.* 2003 Nov 1;362(9394):1445-9.

[38] Brown KA, Offit PA. Rotavirus-specific proteins are detected in murine macrophages in both intestinal and extraintestinal lymphoid tissues. *Microb Pathog*. 1998 Jun;24(6):327-31.

[39] Siemes H, Siegert M, Hanefeld F. Febrile convulsions and blood-cerebrospinal fluid barrier. *Epilepsia*. 1978 Feb;19(1):57-66.

[40] Hall GA, Parsons KR, Bridger JC, Ghatei MA, Ying YC, Bloom SR. Plasma enteroglucagon and neurotensin levels in gnotobiotic calves infected with enteropathogenic and non-enteropathogenic viruses. *Res. Vet Sci*. 1985 Jan;38(1):99-103.

[41] Theoharides TC, Zhang B. Neuro-inflammation, blood-brain barrier, seizures and autism. *J. Neuroinflammation*. 2011 Nov 30;8:168,2094-8-168.

[42] Antonelli T, Ferraro L, Fuxe K, Finetti S, Fournier J, Tanganelli S, et al. Neurotensin enhances endogenous extracellular glutamate levels in primary cultures of rat cortical neurons: Involvement of neurotensin receptor in NMDA induced excitotoxicity. *Cereb Cortex*. 2004 Apr;14(4):466-73.

[43] Shulkes A, Harris QL, Lewis SJ, Vajda JE, Jarrott B. Regional brain concentrations of neurotensin following amygdaloid kindled and cortical suprathreshold stimulation-induced seizures in the rat. *Neuropeptides*. 1988 Feb-Mar;11(2):77-81.

[44] Weclewicz K, Svensson L, Kristensson K. Targeting of endoplasmic reticulum-associated proteins to axons and dendrites in rotavirus-infected neurons. Brain Res Bull. 1998 Jul 1;46(4):353-60.

[45] Shaw DP, Morehouse LG, Solorzano RF. Rotavirus replication in colostrum-fed and colostrum-deprived pigs. Am J Vet Res. 1989 Nov;50(11):1966-70.

[46] Saulsbury FT, Winkelstein JA, Yolken RH. Chronic rotavirus infection in immunodeficiency. *J. Pediatr*. 1980 Jul;97(1):61-5.

[47] Ruiz MC, Cohen J, Michelangeli F. Role of Ca2+in the replication and pathogenesis of rotavirus and other viral infections. *Cell Calcium*. 2000 Sep;28(3):137-49.

[48] Michelangeli F, Ruiz MC, del Castillo JR, Ludert JE, Liprandi F. Effcct of rotavirus infection on intracellular calcium homeostasis in cultured cells. *Virology*. 1991 Apr;181(2):520-7.

[49] Kawashima H, Inage Y, Ogihara M, Kashiwagi Y, Takekuma K, Hoshika A, et al. Serum and cerebrospinal fluid nitrite/nitrate levels in patients with rotavirus gastroenteritis induced convulsion. *Life Sci.* 2004 Jan 30;74(11):1397-405.

[50] Rodriguez-Diaz J, Banasaz M, Istrate C, Buesa J, Lundgren O, Espinoza F, et al. Role of nitric oxide during rotavirus infection. *J. Med. Virol.* 2006 Jul;78(7):979-85.

[51] Borghan MA, Mori Y, El-Mahmoudy AB, Ito N, Sugiyama M, Takewaki T, et al. Induction of nitric oxide synthase by rotavirus enterotoxin NSP4: Implication for rotavirus pathogenicity. *J. Gen. Virol.* 2007 Jul;88(Pt 7):2064-72.

[52] Hagbom M, Istrate C, Engblom D, Karlsson T, Rodriguez-Diaz J, Buesa J, et al. Rotavirus stimulates release of serotonin (5-HT) from human enterochromaffin cells and activates brain structures involved in nausea and vomiting. *PLoS Pathog.* 2011 Jul;7(7):e1002115.

[53] Moon S, Wang Y, Dennehy P, Simonsen KA, Zhang J, Jiang B. Antigenemia, RNAemia, and innate immunity in children with acute rotavirus diarrhea. *FEMS Immunol Med Microbiol.* 2012 Apr;64(3):382-91.

[54] Tian P, Ball JM, Zeng CQ, Estes MK. The rotavirus nonstructural glycoprotein NSP4 possesses membrane destabilization activity. *J. Virol.* 1996 Oct;70(10):6973-81.

[55] Morris AP, Scott JK, Ball JM, Zeng CQ, O'Neal WK, Estes MK. NSP4 elicits age-dependent diarrhea and ca(2+)mediated I(-) influx into intestinal crypts of CF mice. *Am. J. Physiol.* 1999 Aug;277(2 Pt 1):G431-44.

[56] Caraballo RH, Cersosimo RO, Espeche A, Fejerman N. Benign familial and non-familial infantile seizures: A study of 64 patients. *Epileptic Disord.* 2003 Mar;5(1):45-9.

[57] Saghazadeh A, Mastrangelo M, Rezaei N. Genetic background of febrile seizures. *Rev. Neurosci.* 2014;25(1):129-61.

[58] Okumura A, Uemura N, Negoro T, Watanabe K. Efficacy of antiepileptic drugs in patients with benign convulsions with mild gastroenteritis. *Brain Dev.* 2004 Apr;26(3):164-7.

[59] Omata T, Tamai K, Kurosaki T. Clinical study of convulsions with mild gastroenteritis. *Nihon Shonika Gakkai Zasshi* (Tokyo). 2002;106:368-71.

[60] Hayashi K, Sakauchi M, Oguni H, Osawa M. Treatment and outcome of infants who have suffered from clusters of convulsions. Shonika Rinsho (Tokyo). 1999;52:63-7.

[61] Ichiyama T, Matsufuji H, Suenaga N, Nishikawa M, Hayashi T. Low-dose therapy with carbamazepine for convulsions associated with mild gastroenteritis. *NoTo Hattatsu.* 2005;37:493-7.

[62] Richardson V, Hernandez-Pichardo J, Quintanar-Solares M, Esparza-Aguilar M, Johnson B, Gomez-Altamirano CM, et al. Effect of rotavirus vaccination on death from childhood diarrhea in mexico. *N. Engl. J. Med.* 2010 Jan 28;362(4):299-305.

[63] Hull JJ, Teel EN, Kerin TK, Freeman MM, Esona MD, Gentsch JR, et al. United states rotavirus strain surveillance from 2005 to 2008: Genotype prevalence before and after vaccine introduction. *Pediatr. Infect Dis J.* 2011 Jan;30(1 Suppl):S42-7.

[64] Tate JE, Panozzo CA, Payne DC, Patel MM, Cortese MM, Fowlkes AL, et al. Decline and change in seasonality of US rotavirus activity after the introduction of rotavirus vaccine. *Pediatrics.* 2009 Aug;124(2):465-71.

[65] Choi UY, Lee SY, Ma SH, Jang YT, Kim JY, Kim HM, et al. Epidemiological changes in rotavirus gastroenteritis in children under 5 years of age after the introduction of rotavirus vaccines in korea. *Eur. J. Pediatr.* 2013 Jul;172(7):947-52.

[66] Dudareva-Vizule S, Koch J, An der Heiden M, Oberle D, Keller-Stanislawski B, Wichmann O. Impact of rotavirus vaccination in regions with low and moderate vaccine uptake in germany. *Hum. Vaccin Immunother.* 2012 Sep 7;8(10).

[67] Yeom JS, Kim Y, Kim RB, Park JS, Seo J, Park ES. Impact of rotavirus vaccination on rotavirus-associated seizures and a related possible mechanism
. Program and abstract, the 63rd annual fall meeting of the Korean pediatric society; Oct 18-19; Seoul. Seoul: The Korean *Pediatric Society*; 2013.

[68] Payne DC, Baggs J, Zerr DM, Klein NP, Yih K, Glanz J, et al. Protective association between rotavirus vaccination and childhood seizures in the year following vaccination in US children. *Clin. Infect Dis.* 2014 Jan;58(2):173-7.

[69] Weinberg GA. Editorial commentary: Unexpected benefits of immunization: Rotavirus vaccines reduce childhood seizures. *Clin. Infect. Dis.* 2014 Jan;58(2):178-80.

Index

B

C

D

F

G

H

I

J

K

L

M

N

O

P

R

S

T